Cries of Crisis

Cries of Crisis

RETHINKING THE HEALTH CARE DEBATE

ROBERT B. HACKEY

UNIVERSITY OF NEVADA PRESS · RENO AND LAS VEGAS

University of Nevada Press, Reno, Nevada 89557 USA
Copyright © 2012 by University of Nevada Press
All rights reserved
Manufactured in the United States of America
Design by Kathleen Szawiola

Library of Congress Cataloging-in-Publication Data
Hackey, Robert B.
Cries of crisis : rethinking the health care debate / Robert B. Hackey.
p.   ; cm.
Rethinking the health care debate
Includes bibliographical references and index.
ISBN 978-0-87417-889-0 (cloth : alk. paper) —
ISBN 978-0-87417-890-6 (ebook)
I. Title. II. Title: Rethinking the health care debate.
[DNLM: 1. Health Care Reform—United States. 2. Health Care
Costs—United States. 3. Health Policy—United States. 4. Insurance,
Health—United States. 5. Malpractice—United States. 6. Nurses—
supply & distribution—United States. WA 540 AA1]

362.10973—dc23   2012017298

The paper used in this book is a recycled stock made from 30 percent
post-consumer waste materials, certified by FSC, and meets the require-
ments of American National Standard for Information Sciences—
Permanence of Paper for Printed Library Materials,
ANSI/NISO Z39.48-1992 (R2002).
Binding materials were selected for strength and durability.

FIRST PRINTING
21   20   19   18   17   16   15   14   13   12
5   4   3   2   1

For my girls—

Meagan, Sarah, and Tacy

CONTENTS

AT THE HEART OF THIS BOOK lies an audacious claim. The underlying assumptions that frame public deliberations over health care reform in America are misguided, and ultimately counterproductive. For decades, reformers used the rhetoric of crisis to build a case for fundamental changes to the American health care system. This view—which was widely accepted by policy makers, health providers, and the news media—painted a dire picture of a health care system teetering on the edge of collapse. The nature of the crisis varied depending on who told the story: for some, rising costs represented the greatest threat, while others pointed to the growing number of uninsured Americans or the spiraling cost of medical malpractice. Despite these differences, each narrative of crisis shared a common theme—policy makers would be forced to act to avert an impending crisis. This assumption, however, offers the wrong diagnosis for what ails the American health care system.

The origins of this book can be traced back two decades to a conference sponsored by the *Journal of Health Politics, Policy, and Law* at Duke University in 1992. One by one, leading scholars in the field declared that after many decades, universal health care reform was now inevitable. The health care crisis now required decisive action. Editorials in the *Journal of the American Medical Association* and other medical journals echoed similar sentiments. News reports also described the passage of health care reform as a foregone conclusion; the only question, it seemed, was the final shape of the reform package. Soon after the conference, I questioned the inevitability of reform in an article in *Polity* titled "The Illogic of Health Care Reform." From my vantage point, the system remained remarkably stable, as both institutional and ideological forces mitigated against reform. My interest in the rhetoric of health care reform deepened when I had the opportunity to contribute a chapter to an edited volume by Roger Cobb and Marc Ross, *Cultural Strategies of Agenda Denial.* My research for this chapter led me to an eclectic collection of political speeches, newspaper articles, and television reports about how opponents framed arguments against health care reform. This literature revealed an interesting puzzle, for while talk of crisis was commonplace in health care reform debates from the late 1960s to the present, it was conspicuously absent from earlier debates over national health insurance. The health care crisis, it seemed, first became a topic of public debate in the late 1960s. Soon after, I became intrigued by how and why debates over health care reform were defined by the language of crisis.

As my interest in rhetoric evolved to include depictions of crisis in televised medical dramas, movies, and advertising, I found myself writing a different book than I had originally intended. My efforts to make sense of the health care crisis led me to explore new literatures in popular culture, critical theory, and the sociology of social problems. With the assistance of several remarkably capable undergraduates at Providence College, I immersed myself in five decades of news stories, political speeches, and public opinion polls about health care reform. I am deeply grateful too for the work of my dedicated research assistants at Providence College from 2002 to 2010—Jennifer ZuWalick, Jessica (Lopes) Zabbo, Mary Kate Dolan, Jennifer Morgan, Kelly Whalen, and Jackie Bishop—each of whom spent many hours hunting down the raw material for this volume. The mountain of news stories, polls, and transcripts they uncovered led me down new and often unfamiliar paths. I am grateful to my current research assistant, Meghan Drees, for her many hours of marketing research to broaden the reach of my book.

My interdisciplinary focus was enriched during my sabbatical leave at Brown University's A. Alfred Taubman Center for the Study of Public Policy and American Institutions in the spring of 2007 and through my participation in Providence College's Interdisciplinary Faculty Seminar in 2009. The IFS provided me with a wonderful sounding board for my ideas and broadened my intellectual horizons. Our seminar explored a common theme, bringing together faculty from eight different disciplines to explore the nature and meaning of freedom. This experience reinforced my desire to write a book about health care reform that would appeal to colleagues in more than one discipline. I am indebted to my colleague Christopher Arroyo, who introduced me to the work of Ludwig Wittgenstein on the philosophy of language. This volume evolved in fundamentally different ways as a result of our conversations.

I am particularly grateful to my colleagues in the Health Policy and Management program at Providence College. Tuba Agartan, Deborah Levine, and Jessica Mulligan each read drafts of my initial chapters, and their feedback was instrumental in improving the readability and coherence of my argument. Working with the University of Nevada Press was a wonderful experience. I sincerely appreciate the support of Matt Becker, my editor, whose continued enthusiasm and belief in this project provided a much-needed spark to finish the manuscript after many years of writing. I am particularly grateful for Annette Wenda's careful copyediting and for Barbara Berlin's creative suggestions to broaden my audience. Jason Harvey created a visually striking dust jacket that captured the message of my manuscript in a way that exceeded my wildest expectations. I was humbled by the remarkably detailed and constructive feedback offered by the anonymous reviews, which helped me to refine and strengthen my initial arguments. Other debts are more personal. After eight years of long nights and weekends dedicated to this manuscript, my wife and daughters are justifiably relieved to see it finished. This book is dedicated to them.

Cries of Crisis

Constructing the Health Care Crisis

The insecurity created by the health care crisis in America gnaws at the American family and at the deepest roots of our society.
—Leonard Woodcock, Committee for National Health Insurance, quoted in Harold Schmeck Jr., "Panel Asks National Health Insurance," *New York Times*, July 8, 1970

There is no denying our system is broken. Millions of Americans struggle each day because they do not have the coverage they need. . . . The United States is home to the finest medical professionals in the world. These professionals are on the front lines of the crisis, witnessing the failings of our country's health care system first hand every day, as ever more Americans suffer physically and financially. —Senator Max Baucus, "Doctors, Patients, and the Need for Health Care Reform"

THE LANGUAGE AND IMAGERY of a health care crisis are now firmly embedded in contemporary politics and popular culture. For decades, warnings of an emerging crisis provided a rationale for widespread changes in provider payments, medical malpractice claims, and eligibility for public health insurance programs. Crisis talk focused public attention on the need to reform the health care system, underscoring both the severity and the urgency of the policy challenges facing decision makers. Advocates of reform turned to the same familiar narratives each time proposals for reform appeared on the policy agenda. As the *New York Times* noted in 1993, "Fired by a sense of crisis, a majority of Americans say they are willing to accept substantial changes in their health-care system, including government price controls, new taxes, and longer waits for non-emergency appointments." This diagnosis underscored the need for fundamental reform rather than "Band-Aid" solutions. As *ABC News* warned viewers a decade later, this crisis "threatens nearly every city, town, and village in America. The danger is our health care system and what it's doing to people without insurance."[1] Dire warnings of impending collapse are now so commonplace in news coverage, political campaigns, and popular culture that it seems odd to describe the health care system in any other way.

To date, the meaning and significance of the health care crisis remain largely unexplored; reformers use the term in a variety of ways and assign different, often conflicting, meanings to it. Language is significant in debates over health care reform because the labels used to describe policy problems are not neutral. Just as patient narratives are vital to accurate clinical diagnoses, policy narratives shape public views about the state of the health care system, leading to specific diagnoses and policy prescriptions. Drawing upon a growing body of work on the political uses of language, this volume embraces a narrative approach to the study of health policy.[2] My goal is not to produce a comprehensive rhetorical history of health care reform, but rather to explore the various meanings attributed to the health care crisis. This book raises important, yet often unasked, questions for advocates of health care reform. How did the health care crisis become a part of our common vocabulary? How did its meaning evolve over time? What are the policy implications of describing the health care system using the language of crisis?

As an organizing concept, the language of crisis shapes how policy makers, providers, and the public *think* about the health care system. The health care crisis is a potent and enduring political symbol, but crisis narratives offer an oversimplified, and ultimately incomplete, story of what ails the American health care system. Crisis talk captures popular discontent and anxiety about changes in the health care system and the larger economy. In the end, however, narratives of crisis represent a flawed strategy for supporters of health care reform. The rhetoric of crisis generates much heat in health policy debates, but it ultimately sheds little light on what to do to fix the system. Upon closer examination, the concept of a health care crisis means so many different things to so many different groups that it has ceased to have any shared meaning at all.

Crisis narratives suffer from internal inconsistencies that undermine their credibility. First, a forty-year crisis is an oxymoron. The problems plaguing the American health care system are chronic, not acute, conditions. Each time reformers warned of an emerging crisis, opponents dismissed or downplayed these concerns. When the predicted collapse did not occur, narratives of crisis suffered from a serious credibility gap. Second, crisis rhetoric poorly reflects the daily experiences of most patients and providers in the health care system. Despite the persistence of crisis rhetoric, most Americans expressed high levels of satisfaction with their health care providers, and most received the services they needed in a timely fashion throughout the "crisis" period. As a result, crisis rhetoric remains unconvincing for the public, despite its short-term political appeal to candidates and elected officials. Third, repeated cries of crisis generated a policy backlash, as opponents offered competing diagnoses that either challenged the existence of the crisis or questioned reformers' prescriptions.

The American health care system has no identifiable "tipping point" that will necessitate action. As early as 1973, Godfrey Hodgson observed that "most of the things that were wrong with American medicine when President Nixon thought the system faced imminent breakdown are wrong with it now." Hodgson's observation still rings true today. Indeed, as Stephen Shortell and Walter McNerney noted in 1990, "It would be tempting to suggest that the U.S. health care system is now in disarray were it not for the fact that it has never really been otherwise."[3] Continuing talk of crisis also raises public expectations that leaders will act decisively to "cure" the problem. The sense of urgency contained in crisis talk is misplaced, because as a patient, the American health care system suffers not from an urgent, acute condition, but rather from multiple chronic illnesses. By their very nature, chronic conditions defy short-term quick fixes. Instead of curing the problems facing the American health care system, we must build public support to manage them. This is a fundamentally different task, which requires a new rhetorical strategy for reformers.

Crisis narratives also face a significant credibility gap with policy makers and the public. Persistent talk of crisis lends a "Chicken Little" character to health care reform debates, as politicians and the press regularly warn the public that the health care system is on the brink of collapse. Each year, costs continue to rise, more Americans find themselves without health insurance, and the demand for nurses continues to grow. To date, however, the American health care system has avoided the catastrophic "meltdown" predicted by crisis narratives. As a result, cries of crisis lack credibility with both voters and key stakeholders. Dire predictions of an impending meltdown also collide with the actual experiences of most Americans. Although more than fifty million people lacked health insurance in 2010, the overwhelming majority of the public (83 percent) were insured. For the past forty years, insured Americans also expressed high levels of satisfaction with their own health providers and their personal experiences with the health care system, despite their concerns about the overall state of the system itself. Public attitudes about the health care crisis are similar to the "Congress problem," in which voters disapprove of Congress as an institution, but routinely give their own representatives high marks. Indeed, "despite years of intense polling, policymakers remain unsure precisely what people are upset about (beyond the impossibility of enjoying ready access to fine care at minimal cost) and what they think would work better."[4]

Framing health policy problems as crises also raises the stakes for policy makers and discourages the adoption of compromise solutions. Joel Best's analysis of how policy makers use war metaphors to build support for tackling policy problems is instructive, for even when public officials declare "war" on social problems such as cancer, crime, or drugs, public interest in grappling with such intractable issues typically wanes over time. The use of war metaphors in policy debates implies that the enemy can be defeated and that the problem can be eliminated through concerted action.[5] If public officials fail to act or their efforts fail to meet public expectations, their inaction may undermine public confidence in the government's ability to enact meaningful health care reform. Failure to address the "crisis" also produces political fallout for elected officials who raise public expectations about the prospects for reform. Past history offers a sobering lesson, for health care reform contributed to an erosion of public support for presidents from Jimmy Carter to Barack Obama who made expanding access to care and controlling costs a cornerstone of their presidential campaigns.

The problems facing our health care system are familiar and have changed little since the early 1970s. Too many Americans still lack affordable health insurance coverage, health care costs continue to burden businesses and families, and rates of medical error and malpractice remain unacceptably high. Health care reform, in short, is "the oldest rerun in American public policy."[6] The widespread use of crisis rhetoric to describe the state of the American health care system has an ironic twist: the very way reformers framed the debate undermined their ability to address the system's glaring weaknesses. By describing the health care system using images of crisis, reformers preempt more accurate and constructive definitions of the problem and circumscribe public debate about reform. In this context, unpacking the origins and meaning of the health care crisis as a political symbol is vital to the future of health care reform in America.

Paging Dr. Wittgenstein

To understand the frustrations and opportunities facing health care reformers in America, we must first understand how we talk about our health care system and how the nature of our public discourse shapes policy choices.

The work of analytic philosopher Ludwig Wittgenstein offers a useful start-ing point to analyze the rhetoric of health care reform. Wittgenstein argued that "philosophical difficulties are produced by our unwitting abuse of exist-ing concepts." When concepts are misused—or, as Wittgenstein notes, when "language goes on holiday"—the resulting conceptual confusion stymies progress.[7] On the one hand, stakeholders often have different interpreta-tions of words, rooted in fundamental political or economic interests. For example, businesses and workers might reasonably disagree about the best route to control health care costs. In other cases, confusion is purposeful, as affected groups seek to distort or discredit the positions of others.

With no commonly accepted definition of a crisis, warnings of an emerg-ing crisis provide a clear example of Wittgenstein's "language gone on hol-iday." For decades, observers in the media and academia decried the poor quality of public deliberation over health care reform. In 1974, for example, the *New York Times* editorialized that "the public debate which was sup-posedly to lead to the enactment of an effective national health insurance system has turned into a sputtering contest of irrelevant and misleading information." Similar concerns resurfaced after the defeat of the Clinton administration's Health Security Act in 1994, as commentators argued that "vigorous discussion of health care reform . . . produce[d] widespread incom-prehension of the issue and foster[ed] public reluctance to embrace any spe-cific proposal for change." Advocates of reform decried the superficial char-acter of public debate and the prevalence of "horse race journalism" in media coverage. As Ted Marmor lamented, "One hoped for more clarity this time, with a president gifted in communication who might have led the equiva-lent of a national teach-in." The complexity of health care reform proposals led reporters to complain that "health policy almost defies simplification," for "the issues are highly technical, and even the language of the discussion has been dictated in Washington by policy experts."[8] Thus, despite intensive coverage of health care reform by the mass media, public understanding of health care reform declined during the debate over health care reform in 1993–94.

Recent debates over health care reform also prompted much hand-wringing among policy makers and pundits. Health care reform debates aroused intense emotions across the nation in 2009 and 2010. Supporters of reform bemoaned the fact that "some people are choosing diatribe and dis-ruption over dialogue and discourse." At raucous town hall meetings hosted by members of Congress, legislators were often heckled or shouted down by angry constituents. The resulting "debates" over health care reform featured "shouting matches that would make Jerry Springer and Geraldo [Rivera] proud," as police were called in to restore order and escort legislators past mobs of angry protesters. The raucous meetings themselves became a symbol of opposition to Democratic reform proposals, as news reports presented vivid images of irate opponents of health care reform shouting down elected officials. In the wake of such "town brawls," many observers pleaded for greater civility in public discourse. Congressional leaders denounced the "ugly campaign" waged by opponents of reform "not merely to misrepresent the health insurance reform legislation but to disrupt public meetings and prevent members of Congress from conducting a civil dialogue." *USA Today* editorialized that a "dishonest debate" characterized discussions of the proposed health care reform bills in Congress and that "rational argument is being drowned out by outrageous fear mongering."[9]

In the wake of withering rhetorical attacks during the summer and fall of 2009, public support for health care reform fell steadily; by late September, fewer than half of Americans expressed support for reform. Drawing upon fears of rationed care and federally sponsored "death panels," opponents warned voters that "ObamaCare" placed the quality and availability of their health care at risk. Although reformers scoffed at the stories told by opponents, such fear-based appeals resonated with the public.

While reformers fumed that debates over health insurance reform failed to focus on the "real issues," such criticisms miss the point. Debates over health care reform are highly complex, jargon-laden affairs. To participate in such debates, policy makers and the public must first decipher scores of acronyms—DRGs, HMOs, HSAs, IPAs, PPOs, SCHIP, to name but a few—and then struggle to weigh competing assumptions, estimates, and projections for various reform plans. The complexity of reform proposals makes it difficult for many policy makers, let alone the general public, to digest the merits of competing reform proposals. Since policy debates are largely a "passing parade of abstract symbols" for most citizens, it makes little sense to deplore the use of symbolic arguments and "sound bites" to define health policy issues. Symbols are important in policy debates because they enable citizens to break down complex issues into understandable terms.[10] The question is not *whether* we should employ symbolic arguments in health policy, but rather *how* to do so in ways that advance public understanding.

Successful health care reform thus rests upon improving the "narrative competence" of policy makers and the public—in short, their ability to understand, interpret, and act upon policy stories.[11] The "crisis" facing the health care system means different things to different groups, as various stakeholders offer competing diagnoses of the crisis to build support for their own preferred policy prescriptions. Businesses, for example, often define the health care crisis in terms of competitiveness and profitability and seek to control the fiscal burden of providing health benefits for workers and retirees. Solutions that transfer risk from employers to employees, however, yield a different diagnosis of the crisis. Advocates for workers and families argue that shifting more responsibility for financing health insurance to employees simply adds more Americans to the ranks of the uninsured. For workers and retirees, the health care crisis is defined by diminished access to affordable, comprehensive health insurance coverage. Although physicians express concerns about both rising costs and the uninsured, over the past three decades the medical profession expressed the greatest concern over the rising cost of malpractice insurance. With no agreement on the nature or causes of each crisis, forging consensus over how to address the health care system's shortcomings remains an elusive goal.

As a result of this conceptual confusion, the language of health care reform has been "on holiday" for decades. Different groups with different agendas use the same words to describe different phenomena. In such cases, language becomes an impediment to solving public problems, for the terms and concepts used in policy discourse mean different things to different groups. For Wittgenstein, the proper treatment for such cases begins with a careful description of how words are used to uncover their "unnoticed misuse." In the case of health care, the roadblocks to reform include not only interest group opposition, but how debates over reform are framed. To get to the root of the system's problems, reformers must first begin with a clear understanding of how the health care crisis is defined, who defines it, and how it is used.

Constructing the Health Care Crisis

For most of the twentieth century, the need for health care reform was not framed as a crisis. Instead, health care reform was defined by narratives of progress. Efforts to enact compulsory health insurance for workers during the Progressive Era described such proposals as the "next great step in social legislation." During the two decades after World War II, reformers both celebrated the strengths of the American health care system and exhorted policy makers to improve the organization and delivery of care for all. Oscar Ewing, a leading adviser to President Truman, captured this "can-do" postwar optimism in 1947, arguing, "We can have more hospitals, more doctors, more dentists, more medical specialists of all kinds. We can provide better health care for all the people of our land." Opponents responded with charges of "socialized medicine" and images of "assembly line" health care during the tumultuous policy debates over national health insurance in the 1940s and, later, during the debate over Medicare in the early 1960s.[12] Policy makers, physicians, and other stakeholders clashed over the proper role of government in the health care system, but the rhetoric of crisis was conspicuously absent from public discourse during this period.

The postwar optimism that fueled the hospital construction boom, investments in health manpower, and the expansion of public health insurance for the poor and aged was grounded in a narrative of progress. When policy makers in the 1940s and 1950s described issues such as the shortage of nurses as "critical," it denoted the importance of an issue, not the existence of an objective crisis. Few policy makers used the term to denote an actual situation or event.

The contemporary health care crisis has its origins in the summer of 1969. At a nationally televised address, Richard Nixon declared, "We face a massive crisis in this area, and unless action is taken, both administratively and legislatively, to meet that crisis within the next 2 to 3 years, we will have a breakdown in our medical care system which could have consequences affecting millions of people throughout this country."[13] The president's diagnosis of an emerging health care crisis signaled the emergence of a new discourse about health care reform. Prior to Nixon's address, reformers acknowledged the need to "fill in the gaps" in the nation's health care system—for example, by extending health insurance to all—but typically framed the need for reform in terms of equity, not necessity. After 1969 talk of crisis appeared regularly in congressional hearings, news reports, and the political platforms of health providers, organized labor, and business groups.

Within a year of Nixon's address, crisis rhetoric dominated public discourse about the health care system. Writing in the *Atlantic Monthly*, Godfrey Hodgson noted that "by 1970, to say that the American health care system was in crisis had indeed become something of a cliché." Conditions previously viewed as problems amenable to incremental reform were instead redefined as crises. In a 1970 article in the *New England Journal of Medicine*, William Kissick described the health care crisis as a "national preoccupation." By 1976 this "preoccupation" was ingrained in the very fabric of American society, as David Kotelchuk observed that "everyone who watches television, reads a newspaper, or needs a doctor knows that this country faces a health crisis."[14] The declaration that America's health care system faced a crisis represented more than simply a change in vocabulary. This new language signaled a shift in attitudes about health care and the health care delivery system among decision makers and the public. By 1970 conditions that were previously accepted as normal—or even desirable—were now viewed as dangerous or dysfunctional.

Lamenting the state of the nation's health care system now seems as commonplace on the campaign trail as candidates' pledges to curtail waste in government, lower taxes, and spur economic growth. As a political issue, the health care crisis has bipartisan appeal and unites strange political bedfellows. Even political archrivals such as Senator Edward M. Kennedy and President Richard M. Nixon, who agreed on little else, found common ground in their belief that the US health care system was in crisis. Despite their sharp political and policy differences, crisis talk united Democrats and Republicans, liberals and conservatives, health providers and purchasers of care. In particular, crisis narratives allowed candidates to demonstrate that they understood the concerns and problems of everyday Americans. As Bruce Kuklick notes in his study of presidential leadership from Herbert Hoover to Richard Nixon, "What mattered in politics was not what a politician achieved, but how the people felt."[15] In the postwar era, symbolic leadership is increasingly important for political success.

Talk of a health care crisis is a staple of presidential politics. All three presidents during the 1970s—Richard Nixon, Gerald Ford, and Jimmy Carter—urged Congress to address the health care crisis by enacting national health insurance, lending a bipartisan flavor to the debate. The health care crisis returned to the center stage of American politics in the 1990s, when the Clinton administration made reforming the health care system its top domestic priority. Over the past decade, all of the leading candidates for the presidency—Bill Bradley, Al Gore, John Kerry, Hillary Clinton, John Edwards, George W. Bush, John McCain, and Barack Obama—emphasized various elements of the health care crisis as core themes of their campaigns. In 2008 crisis talk defined public debate over health care reform and spanned the political spectrum. In the Democratic primaries, John Edwards—who made health care reform a centerpiece of his 2008 presidential bid—declared that "the American health care system is broken for too many of our families. To fix this crisis, we don't need an incremental shift, we need a fundamental change." Republican candidates sounded similar alarms. Senator John McCain called for immediate action, warning voters, "We are approaching a 'perfect storm' of problems that if not addressed by the next president will cause our health care system to implode."[16]

The language and imagery of crisis have also framed media coverage of health care reform in recent decades. As the *New York Times* noted in 1970, "The manner in which Americans get their health care has been called a nonsystem, a crisis system, and a mess." Media coverage influences the social construction of public problems, for by focusing on certain issues and not others, reporters decide what is newsworthy. In defining what's "news," reporters follow predictable routines that favor certain news stories and concerns. Stories about the state of the nation's health care system are attractive for television reporters because they address a familiar issue. Most Americans utilize health care services in the course of the year, and stories of citizens who cannot afford care, or who receive inadequate care, provide visible victims that attract viewers. The principal characters in narratives about the health care system and its problems—doctors, hospitals, nurses, and patients—are also readily accessible to reporters. Personal stories of the uninsured, or small businesses struggling with rising health care costs, offer engaging "human interest" narratives for readers and television viewers. In 1990, for example, viewers of *CBS This Morning* learned of "a health care crisis here in the city of Chicago," where "more than 600,000 people in the Chicago area have no medical insurance whatsoever. . . . These are people who find themselves being abandoned by a medical system that may, itself, be in critical condition."[17]

Television news reporting places issues in context for the audience by not only describing events, but also analyzing their meaning and significance. News coverage also plays an important role in setting the nation's policy agenda, for policy makers regard news coverage as an indicator of public sentiment and concern. By 2002 the *New York Times* warned readers that "the health care crisis is spreading up the income ladder and deep into the ranks of those with full time jobs" and noted that "the United States is once again confronting a crisis in its health delivery system." News coverage of the emerging crisis emphasized the worsening condition of the nation's health care system. In the weeks before the 2004 elections, the *Des Moines Register* editorialized, "The U.S. health-care system is in crisis. People need help." The message—either implicit or explicit—in such stories of crisis is that dramatic action is needed to avert catastrophe. Similarly, the editors of *USA Today* described the health care system as "an expensive, chaotic mess" in 2006 and warned readers that it "appears dead certain to turn into an all-out crisis."[18]

Televised medical dramas also provide a virtual health education "curriculum" for audiences and reach a wider audience than traditional news outlets such as newspapers, cable news, or documentaries. Popular culture can be an agent of social change by increasing public awareness about emerging issues. Public frustrations with rising health care costs, for example, became a staple of television medical dramas over the past two decades. From caring for the uninsured to medical malpractice, narratives of crisis appeared with growing frequency on popular television dramas. Tens of millions of viewers learned about the struggles of uninsured families by tuning in to episodes of *ER, Chicago Hope, Grey's Anatomy,* and *Scrubs.* Television dramas personalize the complex issues in health care reform debates through familiar characters and story lines. Surveys of *ER* viewers, for example, found that knowledge about health issues such as the human papillomavirus and emergency contraception increased substantially following episodes containing vignettes about each topic. In particular, more than half of viewers reported discussing the health issues addressed on the show with family and friends, and one in seven viewers contacted a doctor or other health provider about a health problem because of something they saw on *ER*.[19]

Portrayals of the health care crisis are not confined to televised hospital dramas. Hollywood movies also dramatized the shortcomings of the American health care system for patients and families through movies such as *The Rainmaker, As Good as It Gets, John Q,* and *Sicko.* Each film grossed millions at the box office, but each also struck a chord with viewers frustrated by rising costs and concerns about diminished access to care. *John Q,* for example, dramatized the plight of a man whose insurance plan refused to cover the cost of a lifesaving transplant for his critically ill son. Media reviews of the films focused much attention on the behavior of audiences—many of whom shouted back at the screen and applauded as characters vented their frustration with rising costs and the restrictive practices of health insurers.[20]

In addition, popular "reality" shows such as ABC's *Extreme Makeover: Home Edition* also highlighted the plight of many uninsured families, as well as families struggling to cope with chronic health problems. Each week, host Ty Pennington introduced viewers to a new family in desperate need of a new home. Families profiled on the show frequently cited the burden of high health care costs as the cause of their current plight. In 2002, for example, the show highlighted the cost of medications for Willie Harvey and his family, who had been unable to afford medication to control his epilepsy prior to the home makeover. Through the show, Willie received a free lifetime supply of medication, along with a stunning new home.[21]

Detoxifying the Debate

Over the past four decades, crisis became *the* lens through which Americans viewed their relationship with the health care system. Indeed, the American health care system suffers from a number of chronic problems. Costs continue to rise at an unacceptably high rate for businesses and families. Medical malpractice remains a major burden for hospitals and physicians. Physicians chafe under restrictive reimbursement systems and new limits on their clinical autonomy, and recurring nursing shortages threaten the quality of care for patients. More than fifty million Americans were uninsured in 2010. Millions more lacked comprehensive coverage, leaving them at risk of substantial out-of-pocket costs in the event of a major illness. While different, efforts to address each of these issues are bound together by a common thread—the rhetoric of crisis.

More than two decades ago, Deborah Stone and Ted Marmor argued that "America remains the most embattled site in the developed world for health policy." Recent debates over health care reform did little to dispel this notion. In the two years after the passage of the Patient Protection and Affordable Care Act (PPACA) (Public Law 111-148) in 2010, a majority of Americans remained confused and conflicted about the bill. Our most recent episode of health care reform reaffirmed that public debates over health care reform lacked not for "new ideas or alternative models," but rather "the ability to put the concepts, ideas, and models together into a package that appeals to a suitably broad cross section of the American public."[22] Doing so remains the principal challenge for advocates of health care reform.

Narratives of crisis offer a flawed rhetorical strategy for achieving this goal. Four decades of crisis talk failed to produce a clear consensus to support the hard choices required to fix what ails the American health care system. Reformers must rework their rhetorical appeals to lay the foundation for meaningful changes that will control costs, expand access to care, and improve the quality of health care provided to all Americans.

The following chapters examine the symbols, stories, and images used to describe the American health care system. Each chapter unpacks the various and often conflicting meanings of the crisis. Chapter 1 provides a conceptual tool kit to analyze the rhetoric of health care reform, drawing on a diverse set of research traditions, including recent studies of rhetoric and public affairs, sociological perspectives on problem definition, and the extensive literature on agenda setting and symbolic politics. In particular, this chapter examines how we came to think about the health care system using the language of crisis. The topical chapters in this volume explore different facets of the health care crisis—rising costs, the high cost of medical malpractice, a shortage of nurses, and millions of uninsured Americans. These competing diagnoses structure how the public came to think about each policy problem as a crisis and how crisis rhetoric frames debates over policy prescriptions. Each chapter also offers an alternative diagnosis that guides reformers away from the cries of crisis toward a more promising path.

The concluding chapter offers a blueprint for redefining public discourse about health care reform. "For democracy to work," Patricia Roberts-Miller observes, "people have to talk. For it to work well, we need to talk well." Debates over health care reform can teach us much about the quality of democratic deliberation in America and, in particular, how policy makers and the public grapple with complex policy problems. To date, health reformers have not "talked well" in debates over how to improve the health care system. By sensationalizing the condition of the American health care system, the rhetoric of crisis diverts attention from meaningful reforms that have the potential to manage, if not cure, the chronic problems we face. Writing in 1993, Lawrence Jacobs noted that the "challenge for reformers . . . is to shape health reform carefully to reflect the enduring meanings that Americans associate with health care and government."[23] To do so, reformers must return to the narratives of progress that framed past debates over health care reform in the 1950s and 1960s. Successful episodes of reform before 1969 built upon core values—equality, opportunity, fairness—to shape public deliberation. No "miracle cure" exists for what ails the US health care system. Instead, the principal task for reformers is to build support for policies capable of managing the long-term, chronic conditions that have plagued the system for decades.

CHAPTER ONE

The Rhetoric of Health Care Reform

To discover our illusions will not solve the problems of our world. But if we do
not discover them, we will never discover our real problems.
—Daniel Boorstin, *The Image*

Words cannot tell us everything we need to know, but they can tell us what we
do not know and what must be discovered.
—Roderick P. Hart et al., *Political Keywords: Using Language That Uses Us*

WRITING IN 1924, Virginia Woolf declared, "On or about December 1910,
human character changed. I am not saying that one went out, as one might
into a garden, and there saw that a rose had flowered, or that a hen had laid
an egg. The change was not sudden and definite like that. But a change there
was, nevertheless; and, since one must be arbitrary, let us date it about the
year 1910."[1] In a similar fashion, the way policy makers, providers, and the
public viewed the American health care system shifted dramatically on or
about 1969. In the span of a few short years, fear replaced progress as the
defining theme in public deliberations over health care reform. Although
President Richard Nixon proclaimed the existence of a health care crisis in
1969, no single triggering event—such as the OPEC oil embargo in 1974 or the
9/11 terrorist attacks in 2001—defined the emerging health care crisis. Nevertheless, the shift in public sentiment was palpable, as characteristics of the
health care system previously regarded as strengths were redefined as weaknesses. Policy makers and the public became preoccupied with rising costs,
the future of the private health insurance system, and the stability and security of their relationships with health providers. By 1970 talk of an emerging
crisis reshaped public sentiments and expectations about the health care
system.

The rapid shift in public sentiment raises several significant questions.
Why did the rhetoric of crisis take root in the late 1960s? What led to such
a dramatic shift in sentiment in such a short period of time? What political, economic, and social circumstances contributed to a growing belief that
the health care system was in crisis? To understand the origins of the health

care crisis in America, we must return to the period before this policy narrative became the principal lens through which Americans viewed their health care system.

Before the Crisis

The optimism and sense of purpose that defined the "American century" were clearly evident in public discourse about health and health care in the 1950s and 1960s. Doctors and medical researchers enjoyed the trust and confidence of the public. Talk of conquering disease was commonplace. The pace of medical progress seemed to be limited only by the availability of resources to fund new research and to make new treatments and therapies available to the general public. As President Harry S. Truman declared in 1947, "There is no more important function of democratic government than to improve the health and increase the well-being of its people." Truman urged Americans to "take action in our common purpose so that each year may bring new victories over disease."[2]

The ascendance of political liberalism in the post–New Deal period also reinforced the notion that in an affluent society, more and better health care was not only possible but achievable. In this context, the principal goal of health policy was to enable more Americans to enjoy the fruits of medical progress. Speaking in 1962, President John F. Kennedy described health as "a prerequisite to the enjoyment of the 'pursuit of happiness.' Whenever the miracles of modern medicine are beyond the reach of any group of Americans, for whatever reason—economic, geographic, occupational, or other— we must find a way to meet their needs and fulfill their hopes." Kennedy left little doubt that achieving this goal was within reach, and he urged Americans to "let this be the measure of our nation."[3]

This powerful sense of optimism was rooted in a faith in scientific progress. By 1960, Godfrey Hodgson notes, "the doctors expected to conquer disease. There was so much publicity about the cure for cancer, the cure for heart disease . . . that people began to feel 'it was only a matter of time before the brilliant, dedicated doctors discovered a cure for death.'" Events in the 1950s reinforced this notion and provided Americans with a palpable sense of the possibilities of modern medicine. A feared killer—polio—was vanquished by a cheap and effective vaccine. Antibiotics became a powerful weapon against infection, and for the first time, new and effective treatments also appeared for patients with common conditions such as cancer and heart disease. Few questioned the notion that disease was curable, or that better health was within reach. By the early 1960s, Americans "believed not in the perfection, but in the perfectibility, of their society."[4]

Truman's efforts to pass national health insurance were stymied by staunch opposition from the medical profession, conservatives, and Republicans in Congress. Fears of creeping socialism framed public debates over health care reform in the 1950s and early 1960s as opponents charged that national health insurance was inconsistent with American values. Nevertheless, progress was palpable. The rapid expansion of private health insurance enabled more Americans to obtain mainstream medical care than ever before. When private, voluntary health insurance plans first appeared in the late 1930s, fewer than four million Americans had insurance to cover the cost of hospital care. A decade later, more than sixty million Americans were covered by some form of health insurance, and news reports predicted that the "spectacular growth" of private health insurance plans would allow most Americans to reap the benefits of medical advances. By 1958 this optimistic appraisal seemed to be borne out, as the number of insured Americans doubled to more than 121 million.[5]

With new medical facilities, more funding for research, and expanded access to health insurance—particularly for those unable to obtain private, employer-based coverage—policy makers seemed confident that the health of the nation would continue to improve. Speaking in 1965, President Lyndon Johnson declared that "we live as beneficiaries of this century's great—and continuing—revolution of medical knowledge and capabilities. . . . The successes of the century are many. The pace of medical progress is rapid. The potential for the future is unlimited."[6] Spending on health care increased steadily during the 1950s and early 1960s, but in an affluent society, good health was seen as a worthwhile investment. In the early 1960s, patients were largely satisfied with the health care system, and with their own relationships with health providers, and merely wanted more—more access, more effective treatments, more cures—in the future. Providers, for their part, were content with a system that imposed few limitations on medical practice, leaving the autonomy and authority of the medical profession unquestioned.

Thus, for two decades after World War II, public deliberations about health policy reflected the aspirations and hopes of the nation. The promise of the "Great Society" articulated by LBJ in the mid-1960s had its roots in a belief in continued social and economic progress. Policy makers and the public shared a common belief that if Americans put their energies into

solving a problem, little could stand in their way. Johnson captured the sentiments of policy makers and the public when he confidently proclaimed that
"we have the power to shape the civilization that we want." In this context,
crisis appeared infrequently, if at all, as a term to describe the state of the
nation's health care system. The few instances in which crisis was used to
label health care issues were linked to an episodic shortage of providers, particularly nurses, during the postwar period. Johnson boldly predicted that
"within your lifetime powerful forces, already loosed, will take us toward a
way of life beyond the realm of our experience, almost beyond the bounds of
our imagination."[7]

Origins of the Crisis

By 1970 Americans' views of the health care system had changed. Everyone—
policy makers, the mass media, providers, and the public—expressed a growing sense of unease with the current state of the health care system. Fears
about the future of the health care system—unheard of ten years earlier—
were commonplace. This change in the rhetoric of health care reform was
particularly evident in the narratives told by policy makers and the press.
The new rhetoric of health care reform reflects the emergence of a new organizing myth to structure public views of the health care system. As Donald
Light observes, "All societies have organizing accounts—what anthropolo-
gists call myths—about the nature of their social institutions, how they came
to their current accomplishments and troubles, and what needs to be done
to overcome these troubles."[8] Myths define the context of policy debates by
providing a set of assumptions about how the world works. The declaration
of a crisis, therefore, reflected a change in public expectations about the
American health care system.

The late 1960s provided a fertile environment for the growth of crisis
narratives. Godfrey Hodgson describes the period from the early 1960s to
the early 1970s as "a time of lost hopes." By the mid-1960s, a growing sense
of public disillusionment was evident across American society. Businesses,
government, medicine, and the professions all faced new scrutiny from a
critical public, as rapidly unfolding events disrupted long-standing relationships. A sense of upheaval defined both foreign and domestic policy debates.
By the end of the decade, Hodgson notes, "the legitimacy of virtually every
institution had been challenged, and the validity of virtually every assumption disputed." This new public mood was evident in declining faith in civic
institutions and the erosion of political trust. In the face of policy setbacks

abroad (for example, the Vietnam War) and at home (integration, race riots, and persistent poverty), Americans began to question the narratives of progress that framed postwar policy making. At the very moment the nation was investing billions of dollars in antipoverty programs and urban renewal, rioting and mass uprisings called into question the ability of government to ameliorate social problems. Talk of crisis replaced confidence as a metanarrative in domestic policy debates as the public was beset by what Rick Perlman describes as "strange new angers, anxieties, and resentments." The shift in public attitudes reflected new doubts about the capacity of government. As Godfrey Hodgson argues, "The real crisis of the sixties was that, for the first time since the civil war and reconstruction, a generation of Americans were compelled to ask not, as people asked in the Depression, how to solve their problems, but *whether* problems could be solved."[9]

In part, the emergence of crisis narratives to describe the state of the American health care system reflected a growing sense of disappointment among patients, providers, and purchasers of care. Disappointment, as A. O. Hirschman argues, is unavoidable, for acts of consumption such as health care services are characterized by a "high degree of variability in . . . quality and efficacy." The passage of Medicare and Medicaid contributed to public unease about the health care system in the mid-1960s. Although both programs afforded millions of Americans access to mainstream medical care, the influx of tens of millions of previously uninsured patients led to significant increases in health care utilization by poor, elderly, and disabled patients. The result, not surprisingly, was longer waits for appointments, rapid increases in the cost of public health insurance programs, and growing concerns about the supply of doctors and nurses to meet the rising demand for health care services. Growing utilization of services thus fanned fears among both publicly and privately insured patients that needed care might not be available, as providers sought to accommodate millions of previously underserved individuals. Ironically, the very success of Medicare and Medicaid planted the seeds of public discontent with the health care system in the late 1960s. Both programs achieved their principal policy goal of increasing access to high-quality health care for millions of underserved Americans. Their success, however, created new fiscal pressures for federal and state governments, as the resulting increases in public expenditures raised concerns about the affordability of government-sponsored health insurance.

Furthermore, while medical advances raised public expectations, additional health care spending often failed to deliver improved health. New treatments for common diseases such as cancer and heart disease, for example, raised public expectations that deadly diseases could be cured. Although overall survival rates improved, for patients and families who failed to respond to the new therapies, the promise of medical progress remained unfulfilled. As Hirschman notes, "In the case of health and educational services . . . performance itself is notably uneven and unpredictable. . . . As a result, the large numbers who lose out in this particular lottery are likely to be an unhappy and disappointed lot."[10]

The economic foundations of narratives of progress—continued economic growth with low inflation that allowed the nation to invest more in domestic and international interests—also began to crumble in the late 1960s. As economic growth slowed, concerns about inflation became widespread. Prices began to rise amid higher spending for the Vietnam War and significant new expenditures for domestic social programs. Inflation had a corrosive effect on both the economy and the national psyche. Concerns about the overall rate of inflation led policy makers and the public to focus renewed attention and scrutiny on health care expenditures, for health care costs outstripped overall prices. In this context, the very programs and policies that were evidence of success in earlier narratives of progress such as improved access to care for the poor and elderly, better pay for nurses and other hospital staff, and the widespread diffusion of new medical technologies and treatments were reinterpreted as causes of inflation.

Economic optimism was also replaced by dire predictions of scarcity, as a growing number of economists and social critics questioned whether future economic growth was possible in the context of limited resources. Scholars warned of the "limits to growth" as a result of resource depletion, overpopulation, and pollution.[11] In this context, additional spending on health was a zero-sum game, consuming resources needed elsewhere in society. Growth in per capita income, which outpaced inflation during the postwar period, slowed by the end of the decade, leading to a decline in real earnings. In an era of rising inflation, the purchasing power of the average American family fell. Continued worries about inflation led President Nixon to impose wage and price controls throughout the economy in 1971.

Finally, the late 1960s marked the end of the liberal consensus that defined domestic policy for much of the postwar period. Although Democrats and Republicans had been unable to reconcile their differences over national health insurance, the two decades after World War II witnessed an extraordinary expansion of federal social programs, including aid to the disabled, health care programs for the elderly and poor (such as Medicare and Medicaid), and a wide range of antipoverty programs. By the mid-1960s, however, conservative opposition to the Great Society and the War on Poverty was growing. The 1966 midterm congressional elections—which handed Democrats their largest electoral setback in a generation—marked a stunning reversal for liberals. In the following years, the rise of the Right was evident in the election of Richard Nixon and in the growing strength of conservatives at the state level (for example, the election of Ronald Reagan to the governorship of California). Party and ideology were also in flux in the late 1960s. By 1968 the New Deal coalition of urban voters, organized labor, and southern whites was fractured by schisms over social policy and the Vietnam War. The rise of the New Left also represented a new challenge for Democratic candidates, as college students and antiwar protesters joined labor and civil rights groups to demand fundamental changes in American society. At the same time, the rise of the Right led to a growing polarization in American politics.

Thus, each of the pillars that supported previous narratives of progress—public confidence in public and private institutions, a strong economy, and a liberal consensus that supported government-led solutions to social problems—had crumbled by 1970. In this climate, crisis narratives soon displaced the stories of progress that had guided reformers since the mid-1940s. Crisis rhetoric drew public attention to larger changes in politics and society. The declaration of a crisis is ultimately a political act that both captures and seeks to direct public sentiment. As Ronald Rotunda notes in his study of political liberalism in America, "Certain symbols, at various times, carry particular significance. In fact, much of United States political history can be interpreted as a rivalry for the possession of certain words."[12] In the 1960s, *crisis* became such a symbol, for it captured a wide range of meanings and experiences. Like all organizing myths, however, narratives of crisis provided an imperfect lens with which to view the American health care system.

The Rhetoric of Crisis

Crisis, as it is employed in public deliberations about health care reform, is an example of what Roderick Hart et al. term a "political keyword." As they observe, all of the words that could be used to describe a problem are not created equal. Instead, "some words are better than others, which is to say, they work harder, get more done, demand more respect. Americans become obedient in the presence of such words." The symbolic power of crisis narratives reflects their ability to capture the fears, insecurities, and anxieties the public brings to debates about health care reform. As a political symbol, *crisis* is familiar to policy makers and the public, for it has been used to frame debates over both domestic affairs (the energy crisis) and foreign policy (the Cuban missile crisis). As *CBS News* anchor Leslie Stahl notes, "The phrase 'America's health care crisis' encompasses everything from large numbers of uninsured to spiraling hospital costs, from outlandishly expensive prescription drugs to a severe and dangerous shortage of nurses."[13] It is, in short, a multipurpose tool that targets Americans' latent fears about the availability, cost, and quality of health care. After four decades, crisis language is now so ubiquitous that any other way of describing the nature of the policy challenges facing the health care system seems suspect.

In health care debates, *crisis* is an example of an "ultimate term." Ultimate terms, as Richard Weaver observes, are abstract concepts or ideas capable of evoking powerful emotional reactions in an audience.[14] Crisis rhetoric is both hierarchical and preemptive, for claims that the health care system is teetering on the brink of collapse represent an effort to "pull rank" on other domestic and foreign policy issues. Using crisis narratives allows reformers to demand public attention and present the public with *the* definition of a problem or issue. Because the public agenda is crowded with many competing issues, this strategy represents a powerful claim for the attention of decision makers.

The ongoing popularity of crisis narratives to frame debates over health care reform is anchored in a belief that stories of impending collapse will force policy makers and the public to take action. "The potency of symbols," as Rebecca Klatch argues, lies "in their ability to instigate action." *Crisis* is an example of a higher-order symbol that conveys a sense of immediacy, regardless of where it is used. Its power depends not on the particular circumstances at a given point in time, but rather on the need for quick and decisive action. As Klatch observes, "Political leaders . . . label a set of events a 'crisis,' connoting a threat or emergency to stir up people's fear, thereby creating the basis for acceptance of particular government actions."[15] In contrast to more situational symbols that refer to events or actors at a specific point in time (for example, "the public option" in debates over health care reform in 2010), higher-order symbols capture enduring images that have broad applicability in a variety of settings. Concepts such as choice, freedom, and liberty reappear in policy debates over time.

The discourse of fear undergirds the narratives of crisis used to describe the American health care system. Whether the topic is the rising cost of health care, the uninsured, the rising cost of medical malpractice, or doctors' relationships with insurers, the common element of all crisis stories is fear. Fears that needed care will be unavailable or unaffordable or that reform will undermine the system's strengths stoked public anxieties. Political leaders have used fear-based appeals such as repeated warnings of an impending "breakdown," "collapse," or "meltdown" to frame each call for health care reform from the 1970s to the present. Beginning in 1969, senior officials in the Nixon administration warned, "This nation is faced with a breakdown in the delivery of health care unless immediate concerted action is taken by government and the private sector." A quarter century later, President Bill Clinton repeated a similar warning, asking Congress to "strike a blow for freedom" by passing health care reform that would enable "Americans to live without fear that their own nation's health care system won't be there for them when they need it." These same fear-based appeals reappeared in 2006, as Senator John Kerry (D-MA) compared the nation's health care system to "a slow-motion [hurricane] Katrina that's ruining lives and bankrupting families all over the country."[16]

News reports also stoked public anxieties about the condition of the American health care system. In a 1993 special report, *CBS News* anchor Dan Rather described the need for health care reform for viewers as "a fear hanging over millions of Americans, the fear of, simply, getting sick. . . . As costs rise, even those who are insured often pay another price in heartache and peace of mind. . . . Tonight, you will share the desperation of families at the very heart of America's health care crisis as they face a terrifying fact of life: the high cost of living also includes the price of just staying alive."[17] Such fearmongering has raw emotional power, as individuals, businesses, and providers worry about the impact of possible changes on both their health and their economic circumstances.

Policy makers and the press personalized images of the health care crisis by presenting the "human face" behind the numbers. The use of synecdoche —representing a larger problem through one person's experience—is also a common feature of crisis narratives. Portrayals of visible victims are regularly used to demonstrate the desperate predicament of families struggling to pay for needed care. A *New York Times* story on the health insurance crisis echoed this same theme in 2002. As one woman quoted in the story worried, "We're eating pancakes some nights as it is. . . . I said to my husband, 'What are we going to do, sell the house so we can pay health insurance?' " Similar horror stories appeared in debates over rising malpractice rates. In 2002, for example, President George W. Bush cited the example of a Nevada physician who left the state after his malpractice premiums rose from $33,000 per year to $108,000 even though he himself had never been sued. Urging voters to support tort reform, the president declared that trial lawyers "have driven this good man out of Nevada."[18]

The endless repetition of fear-based narratives has a cumulative effect, raising anxieties among viewers and readers. For example, dire warnings of doctors driven from practice, or forced to relocate to less costly states, defined each debate over malpractice reform since the 1970s. In 2003 *Today* cohost Matt Lauer introduced a report about medical malpractice with an ominous warning: "For many Americans, the health care crisis in this country does not involve whether or not they have insurance, but whether their doctors can afford to stay in business. Medical malpractice lawsuits are forcing many doctors to close up shop or move out of state." Later that year, the president-elect of the American Medical Association (AMA) warned that as a result of rising malpractice costs, "not only are people deciding not to go into ob-gyn, they're deciding not to go into medicine. The whole profession is at risk."[19]

The Uses and Abuses of Crisis Talk

Crisis narratives serve several important functions in debates over health care reform. First, the language and imagery of crisis enable political leaders and interest groups to communicate complex issues to various publics with differing levels of interest and involvement. In particular, crisis narratives place changes in the health care system such as the rising cost of health care in a larger social context. As Thomas Langston observes in his discussion of presidential rhetoric, "Because events in politics, as in the rest of life, never come with their meanings inscribed on them, people expend a great deal of time and effort trying to figure out what events mean. In doing so, they not only interpret the significance of things that just somehow happened; they in a real sense create, by defining, the events themselves." Crisis stories offer both an explanation for current policy dilemmas and a policy prescription for the public that underscores the need for private sacrifice on behalf of the common good. As Murray Edelman observes, the existence of a crisis is not linked to a specific event, but rather depends on whether decision makers, the mass media, and the public accept it as one.[20]

Policy debates revolve around storytelling. Stories enable voters and citizens to connect abstract issues to their daily lives and simplify complex problems. To understand the challenges facing health care reformers, it is essential to unpack the structure of the stories we tell about the health care system and its problems. The task of rhetoric, after all, is the "study of misunderstanding and its remedies" that is based on a "persistent, systematic, detailed inquiry into how words work."[21] To do so, we must begin by identifying the key elements of the policy narratives used to frame public deliberation over health care reform.

After the failure of health care reform in 1994, political scientist Dan Beauchamp wrote that health care reform "can succeed only if it succeeds as a story, a story about the struggle of the public and the people to have their interests and needs met in a democratic society." Some narratives wistfully evoke a world gone by, while others create optimistic forecasts about a bright future. These may "focus on an older world that is fading into the past" or look to the future by "projecting Utopian visions of ease and abundance."[22] Health policy emerges from the interplay of competing dramatic narratives, each with its own dramatis personae, setting, and intended audience.

The policy-making process is ultimately a conversation about different values and ideas about how the world works. By employing certain words and phrases—in short, by using symbolic appeals—policy makers, interest groups, and the mass media shape how the public views proposals for health care reform.[23] Stories identify the nature and origins of the problems facing the American health care system and offer prescriptions to fix them. Although policy stories and symbols cannot capture all of the nuances of health policy issues, the stories we tell present the public with different ways of understanding the world, leaving citizens to decide for themselves which ones are most credible and persuasive.

Public deliberation about health care reform, therefore, is an example of what Walter Fisher terms "public moral argument." People assess the stories told by the news media, by politicians, and in popular culture by whether they "make sense." Average citizens may lack detailed knowledge about policies and politics, but as "narrative beings" they are nevertheless able to evaluate the credibility and persuasiveness of different policy stories. Fisher argues that all citizens have an "inherent awareness of narrative probability, what constitutes a coherent story, and their constant habit of testing narrative fidelity, whether or not the stories they experience ring true with the stories they know to be true in their lives." Citizens employ a variety of tools to assess the truth-value of the narratives they experience, from personal experiences to television news reports, op-ed pieces, and features on popular talk shows. The narrative coherence of policy stories refers to whether accounts "hang together" without contradictions, while narrative fidelity measures the "truth qualities" of a story by examining the "soundness of its reasoning and the value of its values."[24]

Cries of crisis in debates over health care reform feature several complementary yet distinct stories of decline. As Deborah Stone notes, a story of decline typically begins with "a recitation of facts or figures purporting to show that things have gotten worse. . . . What gives this story dramatic tension is the assumption, sometimes stated and sometimes implicit, that things were once better than they are now, and that the change for the worse causes or will soon cause suffering."[25] Crisis narratives promised supporters of health care reform a short-term political advantage by demanding immediate attention from policy makers. In the absence of a "meltdown," however, repeated warnings of impending collapse were unpersuasive. In the end, narratives of crisis are counterproductive, for their rhetorical shortcomings offer ample opportunities for opponents to challenge, if not discredit, the need for significant policy changes. The result, too often, has been stalemate.

The following chapters explore public deliberation about health care costs, medical malpractice, the nursing shortage, and the uninsured over the past four decades. Each chapter analyzes the emergence of crisis talk and unpacks the rhetorical tools and strategies used to frame debates over health care reform. My goal is to cut through the conceptual clutter that characterizes contemporary debates over health care reform. By understanding the shortcomings of existing narratives of crisis, reformers will be able to tell better and more persuasive stories. As Walter Fisher argues, "The most persuasive, compelling stories are mythic in form, stories of 'public dreams' that give meaning and significance to life."[26] To date, the narratives of crisis that defined our public discourse about health care reform failed to do this.

Four decades of crisis talk is enough. Instead, reformers must seek to capture the public imagination. As Bruce Kuklick observes in his discussion of presidential leadership, "What mattered in politics was not what a politician achieved, but how the people felt. They demanded not that their goals be realized but that their hearts should react in a certain way." Those who seek to cure the health care system must convince policy makers and the public that reform not only is needed, but also represents the next chapter of the American story. The principal challenge for reformers, therefore, is not the development of an ideal plan. Their task is much more fundamental, and hence more difficult. Effective treatments for the chronic problems facing the American health care system must begin by persuading Americans "that the world made sense, that the state had moral authority."[27] In the end, the future of health care reform lies in convincing the public that progress is possible, and that government must be a part of the solution.

CHAPTER TWO

The Cost Crisis

If we're not going to control health care costs, you can forget about controlling the deficit, forget about America being competitive in manufacturing, and forget about restoring our health.
>—Bill Clinton, "Bill Clinton Speaks to Supporters in
>Battle Creek," *CNN*, August 20, 1992

The cost of our health care is a threat to our economy. It's an escalating burden on our families and businesses. It's a ticking time bomb for the federal budget. And it is unsustainable for the United States of America.
>—President Barack Obama, "Transcript of Address
>to the 2009 Annual Meeting of the AMA House of Delegates"

FOR DECADES, public officials and the news media described health care costs using the language of crisis. Reports that health care costs were "exploding," "skyrocketing," or "surging" fanned public alarm. Debates over health care costs reflect broader economic anxieties in American society. Businesses regard the cost of health insurance as an ongoing threat to their productivity and profitability. Crisis talk reinforced the notion that rising costs presented an imminent threat to America's economic well-being. Variations of this same crisis story defined each public debate over the containment of health care costs since the early 1970s.

Such narratives of a looming crisis are familiar but represent only one face of American attitudes toward health care costs. Despite the ubiquity of crisis talk among health reformers and the mass media, a different policy narrative appeared during each debate over controlling health care costs from the 1960s to the present day. In this alternative diagnosis, additional spending on health care is a social choice, not a crisis. Policy makers, providers, and the public regard spending on health care as a worthwhile investment and worry about the consequences of cost controls. In short, higher health care costs are the price of medical progress. From this vantage point, the "side effects" of limiting spending—job losses, limits on the use of promising new therapies, and slowing the search for new cures—would be far worse than the disease itself.

The difficulty of controlling health care costs in America is rooted in these dueling narratives. Public deliberation about health care spending illustrates what Wittgenstein describes as the "unwitting abuse of existing concepts," for after four decades of crisis talk, the meaning and significance of increased spending on health remain in dispute. Our inability to make hard choices about whether, and how, to limit the cost of health care mirrors the two faces of health care spending—in which rising costs are regarded as *both* a crisis and an investment. As a result, cost containment continues to be an elusive goal.

As a political symbol, the cost crisis illustrates the importance of attributed meaning in framing social problems. Talk of a health care cost crisis thus raises more questions than it answers. How, for example, should the scope and incidence of the cost crisis be measured? Should policy makers focus on health care's share of the larger economy (for example, the gross domestic product [GDP])? Or should they seek to reduce the rate of increase in health care spending? If the latter, should policy makers focus their attention on insurance premiums? Hospital charges? The price of pharmaceuticals? Four decades of crisis talk, in short, created a conceptual thicket for public discussion of cost containment.

Since the public views spending on health care as both a bane and a blessing, policy debates are fraught with inconsistent, often contradictory, expectations. As purchasers of care, individuals and businesses support efforts to control costs, but as potential consumers of health care services, they remain wary of proposals that would limit their access to the latest medical treatments. Furthermore, the patients and policy makers continue to support additional investments in medical research.[1] In the long run, these policies result in higher spending, as new technologies such as diagnostic imaging, pharmaceuticals, and personalized medicine often supplement rather than replace existing treatments. Americans remain wary of explicit, "painful" prescriptions to control costs. In the absence of a consensus over what to cut, the prospect for meaningful cost containment is dim. Thus, the principal challenge for health care reformers lies not in the development of policy tools, but rather in forging a consensus over the need for cost containment in the first place.

The unnoticed misuse of language hinders public discussions of cost containment in several ways. First, continued cries of a cost crisis lack traction with the public. At no point during the past four decades did the health care system reach a tipping point where additional spending led to economic collapse. The persistence of crisis talk, however, led defenders of the status quo to challenge both the diagnosis and the policy prescriptions offered by reformers. Each time proposals for significant cost containment appeared on the policy agenda, critics argued that the "crisis" was either overblown or nonexistent. When rising costs do not lead to an economic meltdown, subsequent warnings of an emerging crisis suffer from a growing credibility gap. Crisis talk misdiagnoses what ails the American health care system, for rising costs are a chronic, not an acute, problem. Second, calls for cost control fail to resonate with the public. Spending on health care services and medical research remains popular with policy makers and the public. In particular, since costs for one group represent income for others, key stakeholders such as doctors, hospitals, and pharmaceutical firms have a limited appetite for "painful prescriptions" such as rationing. Crisis rhetoric is also poorly suited to frame debates over cost containment, which is ultimately an exercise in priority setting. Rising costs are a long-term secular trend not only in the American health care system, but in those of other industrial democracies. As a chronic condition, health care inflation cannot be cured, but rather must be managed. To do so, policy makers must engage the public in serious conversations about what forms of health care spending generate the most value and what, if any, limits should be placed on the use of new technologies and treatments.

Narratives of Crisis

The same narratives of crisis and familiar symbols and stories of progress structured how the media, policy makers, and the public talked about health care costs since the late 1960s. First, fear framed media coverage and political debates over health care spending. Fear-based narratives painted a picture of a growing problem that affected individual families, organizations, and the larger society. As a result, rising health care costs captured middle-class anxieties about global competition, stagnant wages, and the threat of job losses. Health care costs burdened visible victims who were familiar to millions of Americans. The principal characters in these stories— hardworking small business owners and workers—were portrayed as innocent victims of rising costs. Thus, the rhetoric of crisis created a powerful symbolic enemy.

Second, talk of a health care cost crisis reinforced the notion that the health care system was fast approaching a breaking point in which current levels of spending on health care could no longer be sustained. Relentless inflation—both in absolute and in relative terms—featured prominently in news stories and political rhetoric. Speaking to the American Medical Association in 1983, President Ronald Reagan described growing spending on health care as "malignant." News reports, political candidates, and business groups described well-managed firms pushed to the brink by rising health care costs. Diagnoses of a cost crisis contain an implicit policy prescription, for they underscore the need for decisive action to rein in "runaway spending." Indeed, President Barack Obama described health care reform as "an economic imperative" in town hall meetings around the nation during the summer of 2009.[2]

Third, crisis narratives underscored the broad reach of rising costs for all Americans. The AARP's monthly magazine, *Modern Maturity*—the largest circulating monthly periodical in the United States—warned readers in 1990 that "every sector of our society is being shaken by the national health care crisis as federal and state governments, insurers, and businesses engage in a frenetic game of hot potato, trying to toss the burden of health care costs to someone else." The cost crisis touched every home: business owners faced lower profits and uncontrollable spending, which were passed along to workers in a variety of ways, from increased cost sharing to lower wages. As *ABC News* reported in 2003, "The problem of higher health care costs is affecting everybody, management as well."[3]

Finally, narratives of crisis evoked bipartisan alarm. Every president from Lyndon Johnson to Barack Obama identified rising health care costs as an important domestic policy problem. Newspaper stories, nightly news programs, and periodic "special reports" on television all reported different variations of the same crisis story: health care costs, whether defined in terms of spending on hospital care, pharmaceuticals, or the overall "slice" of the economic pie, were spiraling out of control. Hollywood also picked up this theme, for movies such as *John Q* and *Sicko* underscored the vulnerability of insured Americans to economic ruin as a result of unanticipated medical costs. Repeated warnings of crisis, however, failed to persuade the public of the need to support cost containment. The health care cost crisis, therefore, is ultimately a matter of perspective. Costs represent not only an economic burden, but also a source of economic growth and hope for patients and families struggling with illness.[4]

Constructing the Cost Crisis

Since 1969 the conventional wisdom in health policy debates portrayed health care spending as an emerging crisis. As *NBC News* reporter Ron Allen informed viewers in 2002, "There is no single issue more contentious in this country than the cost of health care."[5] The crisis was framed by stories of decline, which warned that rising costs threatened the continued profitability of businesses and, by extension, the economic well-being of workers. Reformers employed vivid images and horror stories to dramatize the significance of the cost crisis for the mass media and the public.

The notion of an emerging crisis in health care costs first appeared in the late 1960s. The new definition of health care costs as a crisis marked a dramatic break with the past image of health care spending. For most of the twentieth century, increased spending on health care was a mark of social progress, not a crisis. Health care expenditures increased steadily during the 1950s and 1960s without being labeled as a crisis. By the mid-1960s, news reports noted that health care costs had tripled since 1950, reaching more than 6 percent of the nation's gross domestic product. Additional spending on health care during this period, however, did not arouse public concern of an impending breakdown in the health care system. Instead, news reports described additional spending as the price of progress: "If we want to bring the highest quality of medical care to the greatest number of people there is no alternative but to pay the costs involved."[6] In an increasingly affluent society, spending more on health care was regarded as a worthwhile investment.

The growth of medical expenditures accelerated during the 1950s and 1960s, as the annual rate of medical care spending rose from 7.5 percent during the period from 1947 to 1957 to 8.4 percent in the decade that followed. After hospital costs rose by 36 percent over a five-year period from 1959 to 1964, academic observers wondered "whether increases of the current order could be absorbed." In addition, health care's share of the American economy—typically expressed as the percentage of the nation's gross domestic product devoted to health—also increased markedly during this period, from 4.5 percent in 1950 to 6 percent in 1965. By the late 1960s, health care costs had outstripped the consumer price index for more than a decade, increasing 170 percent from 1960 to 1970.[7]

Following the passage of Medicare and Medicaid in 1965, rising costs generated a growing sense of alarm. By 1967 even steadfast supporters of reform such as Senator Robert F. Kennedy (D-NY) described the cost of health care in America as "staggering . . . more than 6% of our gross national product." For liberal reformers who viewed Medicare and Medicaid as the first step toward universal coverage, rising costs threatened the future prospects of national health insurance. The spiraling cost of public health insurance programs, however, was cited by conservatives as evidence of an out-of-control welfare state. As the 1960s drew to a close, news reports described "spiraling" hospital costs as the "No. 1 subject for discussion" among patients, physicians, and hospital administrators. Spurred by reports that hospital charges had doubled over the previous decade, five different congressional committees held hearings on the rising cost of health care in 1968. Later that year, Senator Abraham Ribicoff (D-CT) proposed to hold "indefinite" hearings to uncover the root causes of health care inflation. A growing sense of alarm—the harbinger of crisis rhetoric in future years—was evident in the testimony before Ribicoff's committee. As one physician warned the assembled senators, "Unless the health care industry takes such steps to instill order in the current chaotic situation, very likely we will experience a series of major breakdowns in the health services system."[8]

Inflation emerged as a major economic policy challenge in the late 1960s, ultimately leading President Richard Nixon to impose national wage and price controls in 1971. This fear of runaway costs provides the context for Nixon's proclamation of an emerging cost crisis in 1969. The president's advisers warned that "a crippling inflation in medical costs" could send a ripple effect throughout the economy. Soon after the president's address to the nation, media reports also embraced the language of crisis to describe rising health care costs. News reports defined higher health care spending as a "grave crisis" and compared the "galloping costs" of health care to "a runaway line on a fever chart."[9] This analogy is telling, for it suggested that health care costs were a treatable, acute condition. To the extent that policy makers and the public embraced this notion, debates about containing health care costs focused on administering short-term fixes—the policy equivalent of aspirin and Tylenol—to bring costs down.

By 1971 talk of crisis was commonplace in Washington, reflecting a dramatic shift in public sentiment about health care costs from the mid-1960s. In his call for a new national health strategy in 1971, President Nixon asked all Americans to "join together in a common effort to meet this crisis." The president underscored the severity of the problems facing the nation's health care system, noting, "Nineteen months ago I said that America's medical care system faced a 'massive crisis.' Since that statement was made, the crisis has deepened." This sense of urgency was also evident in Congress, as Senator Richard Schweiker (R-PA) declared, "We all know the health care crisis is very severe."[10]

Concerns about inflation kept health care spending on the front burner of the nation's policy agenda during the 1970s. By 1976 the average American family spent more than one-ninth of its earnings on health care, and health care costs outpaced both workers' earnings and the consumer price index. As the *New York Times* observed, "Two of the rites of spring in Washington are the arrival of tourists to view the cherry blossoms and the sending to Congress of the Presidential health message containing hard facts about rising health care costs and tough rhetoric demanding action to brake them." Each president promised swift and decisive action to bring costs under control. In 1977 President Jimmy Carter noted, "Expenditures on health care have been rising at an extraordinary rate. Since 1950, the cost of health care has risen 1,000 percent." As a result, the president warned that "the cost of [health] care is rising so rapidly it jeopardizes our health goals and our other important social objectives." As the 1970s drew to a close, the *New York Times* editorialized that "everyone agrees that something has to be done to control exploding medical costs." Vice President Walter Mondale observed that "health care costs are rising—this is sheer inflation—at the rate of $1 million per hour, 24 hours a day, and has [*sic*] been doing so now for several years." Hospital industry officials worried that "if we don't govern health care costs, we will contribute to the destruction of the free enterprise system." In an effort to forestall government price controls, providers pledged to undertake a "voluntary effort" to control spending on health care costs in 1979.[11] Nevertheless, health care costs continued to soar.

Reformers used similar stories of decline—and metaphors—to warn the public about rising costs in the 1980s. In a remarkable turn reminiscent of Nixon's wage and price controls, the Reagan administration—elected on a platform of limited government—turned to price controls for inpatient hospital services as a means of reining in runaway Medicare and Medicaid costs. The resulting legislation—the Tax Equity and Fiscal Responsibility Act of 1982—transformed the way doctors and hospitals were paid for inpatient care from a retrospective, cost-based system to a prospective payment model that limited the autonomy of both physicians and hospital administrators. Nevertheless, former vice president Walter Mondale warned that the "unbelievable runaway costs of health care" were a "disaster" during his 1984 presidential bid. In a similar vein, the secretary of health and human services, Margaret Heckler, described rising costs as a "health care inflation monster that has plagued us for more than two decades."[12]

Media coverage also emphasized the urgency of the crisis. Television news coverage, in particular, introduced millions of Americans to its scope and impact. In 1991 CBS coanchor Charles Osgood described "the rapidly growing cost of health care ... [as] a national crisis." Vivid descriptions of rising costs featured prominently in news stories about health care spending. As *CBS News* health reporter Dr. Bob Arnot declared, "You won't get much of an argument if you say that health care costs are spiraling out of control." To bring the issue home for viewers, Arnot noted that "Americans spend $23,000 a second on medical care. That's more than $2 billion a day, $733 billion a year, an increase of 100 percent in just five years."[13]

Public discourse about health care costs remained frozen in time from 1969 to 2010. Warnings of impending collapse—and the need for decisive action—reappeared in each debate over cost containment. By 1990 Senator Jay Rockefeller (D-WV)—one of the cochairs of the bipartisan Pepper Commission—declared that "the American health care system is in total crisis. We're plunging ahead in this country toward a health care catastrophe." As Senator Bob Kerrey (D-NE) warned in 1991, "Increases in cost ought to alarm all of us." He predicted that "it'll be three or four years before that cost collapses the system and causes the citizens to want to do something." Similar predictions of an impending meltdown reappeared during recent debates over health care reform. By 2007 economist Laurence Kotlikoff argued that the health care system had reached a "suicidal status quo" that was "driving the country to fiscal, financial, and economic ruin." The United States, he argued, "has been pumping more and more air into an already overinflated tire and there is a point at which it will burst, unless the pressure, particularly in the area of healthcare spending, is released." Soon after taking office, President Barack Obama also invoked the rhetoric of crisis to mobilize support for health care reform. The president declared the health care system was "breaking America's families, breaking America's businesses, and breaking America's economy." Christine Romer, a leading economic adviser for the Obama administration, sounded a similar alarm. Romer warned, "The one thing that's happened relative to the 1990s is the nightmare scenario is getting closer."[14]

Media reports on health care costs also underscored the urgency of the cost crisis. As *Newsweek* warned readers in 2009, "The U.S. health care system is on an unsustainable path. If current trends continue—and there is no indication that they won't—health care will consume 40% of the national economy by 2050." As Congress undertook serious debate over health care reform in 2009, *USA Today* editorialized that "medical costs are rising so fast that they threaten to double premiums in about a decade, and bankrupt the country later on, so doing nothing isn't a viable option." Senator Olympia Snowe (R-ME) emerged as a central figure during the debate over health care reform in Congress in the fall of 2009. The day after casting the only Republican vote in support of Senator Max Baucus's (D-MT) "bipartisan" reform plan, Snowe was interviewed on *Today*. She explained her vote by noting the urgency of the situation. "Given the historic rise in health care costs it's on the short term horizon that we're going to have a serious crisis." Snowe compared passing health care reform to "turning the Titanic around before it hits the iceberg. That's the situation we're finding ourselves in today with rising health care costs. It's going to put the health care system into a death spiral. We know that it's putting it out of reach for Americans and for employers."[15]

An Unsustainable Burden for Employers

The notion that rising health care expenditures threatened the economic competitiveness of American firms and, by extension, of the larger economy gained widespread acceptance in the 1970s and soon became the conventional wisdom in health policy debates. In this narrative, the burden of health care costs can be felt across the nation in lost jobs and lower profits.

Crisis narratives were particularly evident in public discourse about the future of the American automobile industry. By the early 1970s, domestic automakers cited spiraling health care costs as a significant threat to their economic competitiveness. News reports noted that automakers spent more on health benefits for unionized workers than they did for the steel used to produce their vehicles. Automakers passed health care costs along to consumers in the form of higher retail prices; in 1975 consumers who purchased a new General Motors (GM) vehicle paid about $160 toward the cost of health insurance for autoworkers and their families. By 1976 the Big Three US automakers spent more than $1.4 billion on health insurance, leading Ford executives to complain that "there is just so much a corporation can cover through its productive efforts. We have reached that point. We want relief."[16]

The following decade brought no relief. For automakers, rising health care costs became a matter of life and death. By the early 1980s, GM officials estimated that the company's health care costs per vehicle had more than doubled since 1974. Industry executives cited their health care costs as a principal reason the Big Three could not compete on an even footing with foreign automakers. At Chrysler health care costs exceeded $400 million in 1984, or $550 for each car it sold; the company had to sell about seventy thousand vehicles to pay for its annual health care costs. The burden of health care costs for current workers and retirees continued to increase throughout the 1980s and by 1991 added $700 to the cost of each vehicle.[17]

Concerns about the cost of health care spurred businesses and political candidates to endorse health care reform in the early 1990s. On the campaign trail in 1991, Senator Bob Kerrey told voters that if the nation failed to bring costs under control, "the rising cost of the current system [will] crimp U.S. businesses' ability to thrive in a world where our major competitors enjoy universal health care at far lower costs." Corporate leaders argued that US firms faced a competitive disadvantage as a result of spiraling health care costs. In this story of decline, rising costs threatened businesses, both big and small. As officials from the National Restaurant Association argued in 1991, "With the health care system structured as it is today, small business cannot really afford to provide health insurance." Senator Jay Rockefeller concurred with this diagnosis, noting that "46% of business profits in this country go to paying the cost of health care. Small business, big business, everybody's drowning under the cost." Soon after taking office in 1993, President Bill Clinton declared that "our medical bills are growing at over twice the rate of inflation, and the United States spends more of its income on health care than any other nation on Earth. And the gap is growing, causing many of our companies in global competition severe disadvantage."[18]

In recent years, the spiraling cost of employer-sponsored health insurance led Wall Street analysts to quip that American automakers had effectively become "HMOs with wheels." In 2004 GM was the nation's largest private purchaser of health care, insuring more than 1 million families at a cost of more than $5.2 billion. The following year, the company reported that its health care costs for workers and retirees had increased by nearly $1 billion in the preceding twelve months—an annual increase of more than 20 percent. The cost of health insurance benefits for current workers and retirees exceeded $1,500 per vehicle. Thus, automakers had become, in effect, "a social insurance system that sells cars to finance itself." The *Wall Street Journal* underscored the urgency of the situation in 2005, editorializing that "these costs are unsustainable now that GM has only one worker for three retirees, and when Honda and Toyota aren't burdened by the same unionized benefit levels in Tennessee and Ohio, much less in Nagoya." Controlling health care costs was essential to the continued viability of the American automobile industry. Writing in 2007, Boston University economist Laurence Kotlikoff declared, "Rising health care costs are driving American companies broke. . . . It's no coincidence that Ford Motor Company is spending over $3 billion per year for healthcare for its retirees and current workers, that those costs are rising annually in real terms at roughly 6 percent, and that it is in the process of laying off 40% of its workforce." Soon after taking office, President Barack Obama observed that "a big part of what led General Motors and Chrysler into trouble in recent decades were the huge costs they racked up providing health care for their workers; costs that made them less profitable, and less competitive with automakers around the world. If we do not fix our health care system, America may go the way of GM—paying more, getting less, and going broke. When it comes to the cost of our health care, then, the status quo is unsustainable."[19]

Media coverage of health care costs also dramatized their impact on business profits. As the *New York Times* noted in 2002, "In a struggling economy, many employers say they can no longer simply absorb these higher costs." News reports defined cost containment as a matter of life or death for businesses, warning that "the most progressive companies understand that their very survival is at stake if they don't get a handle on their health care costs." The cost crisis offered reporters a powerful human interest story. News reports personalized the toll of rising costs on small businesses, bringing viewers "behind the scenes" to see the havoc wreaked by rising health insurance costs. As *ABC News* reporter Jackie Judd noted in a 2003 story, "When Harold Goldmeier took over the family business in Chicago twenty two years ago, health insurance for his employees was completely affordable. Today it's a back breaking expense. . . . Goldmeier even had to stop paying for employees' family members." Since three-quarters of American companies employ twenty or fewer workers, the problem of rising health care costs is a proximate issue for millions of Americans. By 2004 the *Wall Street Journal* reported that "after four years of double-digit growth—at a time when the general inflation rate in the US is 3%—the cost of providing health care, particularly to employees' family members, is fast becoming unaffordable for many companies."[20]

Corporate leaders issued dire warnings about the cost of inaction. As the CEO of Wal-Mart declared in 2006, "The soaring cost of health care in America cannot be sustained over the long term by any business that offers health benefits to its employees. And every day we do not work together to solve this challenge is a day that our country becomes less competitive in the global industry." In an employer-based health insurance system, rising costs threatened to unravel benefits for millions of American families. After taking office in 2009, President Barack Obama stressed the importance of cost

control with similar stories of decline. "Costs," Obama declared, "are hurting business, as some big businesses are at a competitive disadvantage with
their foreign counterparts, and some small businesses are forced to cut benefits, drop coverage, or lay off workers."[21]

Congressional supporters of health care reform also described controlling
health care costs as an economic imperative. Senator Max Baucus noted,
"Small businesses across the country do the math and conclude they have
no choice but to cut health benefits for their employees because premiums
have simply become unaffordable." Urging his colleagues to support a compromise on health care reform, Baucus reminded lawmakers that "over the
past decade, American families and businesses have seen their costs sky-
rocket. Today, employer-based coverage for a family of four typically costs
more than $13,000. . . . Our current system is simply unsustainable." Support-
ers of reform—including labor leaders and the CEO of Wal-Mart—urged policy makers to "remove the burden that is crushing America's businesses and
hampering our competitiveness in the global economy." This same argument
was echoed by the US secretary of commerce, who warned, "Rising health
care costs are crushing American companies—particularly small businesses
that are the source of much of our economic vitality. . . . Costs rising at this
rate are unsustainable and put U.S. firms at a competitive disadvantage to
foreign companies. . . . It also destroys U.S. jobs."[22] In this narrative, rising
health care costs affect all Americans.

In a related story of decline, reformers noted that rising costs contributed
to stagnant earnings and fewer job prospects for American workers. As Bill
Clinton declared in 1993, "The average American worker would be making
$1,000 a year more today if health care accounted for the same proportion
of wages and benefits as in 1975. Unless we act, health care costs will lower
real wages by almost $600 per year by the end of the decade and nearly one
in every five dollars Americans spend will go to health care." A decade later,
Senator John Kerry (D-MA) declared that "it's wrong to allow skyrocketing
health care costs to choke off new jobs, eat up family incomes, and leave millions uninsured." Similar stories of decline reappeared in 2009, as President
Barack Obama told the nation that "I don't accept a future where American
business is hurt and our government goes broke. . . . With each passing year,
health care costs consume a larger share of our nation's spending and contribute to yawning deficits we cannot control." Speaking before the American Medical Association, Obama warned that "if we fail to act, one out of

every five dollars we earn will be spent on health care within a decade. In thirty years, it will be about one out of every three—a trend that will mean lost jobs, lower take home pay, shuttered businesses, and a lower standard of living for all Americans."[23]

A Second Opinion: The Price of Progress

Despite repeated cries of crisis, a different perspective on health care costs challenged this conventional wisdom each time proposals for cost containment appeared on the public agenda. This alternative diagnosis struck a responsive chord with policy makers, patients, and the public, for it tapped into deep-seated American values. Both providers and patients pointed to the fruits of continued medical innovation and progress that paid dividends in the form of longer lives, improved treatments, and better quality of life for millions of Americans. Opponents of reform also noted that spending on health care contributed to economic growth and warned that overly aggressive cost-containment policies could hinder job creation. Finally, critics contended that efforts to control spending on health care would interfere with the creativity of the marketplace, limiting the availability of potentially lifesaving therapies and treatments. Health care, in this narrative, was a sound investment.

For most of the twentieth century, additional spending was hailed as a mark of success, not as a sign of a system in distress. Concerns about the rising cost of hospital care were evident in the early 1960s, but the rhetoric of crisis was conspicuously absent from public discourse. In the decade before Nixon's declaration of a health care crisis, the price of health care outstripped the overall cost of living in both absolute and relative terms. This fact, however, did not lead policy makers or the public to conclude that the nation was spending too much for health. For two decades after World War II, Americans expressed confidence in the ability of modern medicine to deliver longer, better-quality lives. As Herman Somers and Anne Somers wrote in 1961, however, "Most Americans do not question the legitimacy of increased spending for health." Additional spending was not seen as a crisis, for "if these additional expenditures buy a commensurate amount of additional health protection, there appears little question that it would represent a justifiable allocation of national resources. The nation could afford it."[24] While policy makers decried "unjustified price increases" by health insurers, hospitals, and other providers, the public did not challenge the fundamental notion of health care spending as a worthwhile investment. This view of health care spending stands in stark contrast to the dire warnings of an impending crisis that appeared in subsequent years.

News reports in the 1960s noted, "If we want to bring the highest quality of medical care to the greatest possible number of people there is no alternative but to pay the costs involved." In this context, the rising cost of health care simply represented the price of medical progress. This view of health care costs has its roots in Americans' long-standing beliefs in scientific and technological progress. During the postwar period, the US health care system fostered the diffusion of expensive medical therapies for the critically ill, from iron lungs and intensive care units for cardiac patients to trauma centers and teaching hospitals. As David Rothman observed, "Americans have an extraordinary romance with medical technology, particularly when it has the capacity to save the almost moribund patient."[25] New treatments enabled physicians to save the lives of patients who suffered from previously incurable conditions. Evidence of medical progress appeared in communities across America, as hospitals across the nation met public demands for new and improved services and the nation's medical schools expanded the health care workforce. The fruits of medical progress—whether in the form of vaccines against feared diseases such as polio or steady progress against heart disease—offered tangible proof that investments in health care saved lives.

Winning the War Against Disease

President Richard Nixon's declaration of "war" on cancer in his 1971 State of the Union address captured the duality of health care spending. On the one hand, Nixon repeated his earlier call to "slow the alarming rise in the costs of medical care." In the same address, however, the president asked legislators to approve "$100 million to launch an intensive campaign to find a cure for cancer." The language of investment was evident in Nixon's promise to "ask for whatever additional funds can be effectively used." Abandoning the talk of a health care cost crisis that had defined his first two years in office, Nixon underscored the historic opportunity facing the nation. Underlying this narrative was a simple yet powerful assumption: if afforded the resources, the medical profession would conquer disease. The principal barrier to medical progress was a shortage of funding, personnel, and facilities, not a lack of knowledge. Nixon declared, "The time has come in America when the same kind of concentrated effort that split the atom and took man to the moon should be turned toward conquering this dread disease." Cost containment was conspicuous by its absence, even though the success of the new research endeavors would invariably generate new, more expensive diagnostic tools and treatments. The president called on all Americans to join in "a total national commitment to achieve this goal."[26] Soon after, Congress unanimously passed a resolution that committed the nation to curing cancer by 1976.

This deadline was not met, and a cure for cancer remains an elusive goal. Nevertheless, the failure to find a cure did not dampen public support for medical research. Instead, calls for additional research funding are based on stories of stymied progress. In such narratives, a "search for the cure" saves lives by developing new treatments and technologies. Conversely, a failure to invest additional money into medical research and treatment places lives at risk. As noted medical sociologist David Mechanic observes, "However jaundiced the medical care experts have become about the excesses, inefficiencies, ineffectiveness, and irrelevance of much of medical care, the fact is that the public does not share this perspective. Increased investment in medical care continues to be highly valued by the public."[27]

In this alternative diagnosis, rising costs reflected the widespread availability of improved lifesaving treatments; health care costs were lower in the mid-twentieth century because doctors had few effective treatments for common health care problems. Following his heart attack in 1957, for example, the principal treatment for President Dwight Eisenhower was bed rest. None of the elements of today's medical tool kit—clot-busting drugs, angiography, open-heart surgery, or imaging tools—were available to the president's physicians. Similarly, when President John F. Kennedy's newborn son Patrick died of respiratory distress syndrome in 1963, no neonatal intensive care units existed to provide lifesaving treatment. Today most newborns with similar conditions survive thanks to advances in neonatology. In recent decades, the pace of medical progress was palpable, and the rapid diffusion of new lifesaving therapies was widely covered in the news media. Although investments in research ultimately led to the development and diffusion of new, costly therapies, few questioned the wisdom of further progress in the war against disease.[28]

A decade after Richard Nixon's declaration of a health care crisis, news reports continued to express a fundamental sense of optimism about the impact of health care spending on the health of the public. "Historically, bigger spending on health care has led to better health. Life expectancy in the 70s is improving four times as fast as in the previous 15 years. Differences in life expectancy between blacks and whites have been cut by a third; infant mortality is down a fifth." In this context, critics dismissed concerns that rising spending would result in economic ruin. Indeed, "of all the major components of our economy, medical care may be the only one in this inflationary era that can justify its costs on the basis of quality. You pay more and you get more.... [A]s the quality of medicine continues to improve we have to expect to pay more for it."[29]

These cases illustrate a fundamentally different side of health care spending. Spending more on health care is a choice, not a crisis. Narratives of progress derive their enduring appeal from the power of hope, for diseases that once ravaged society—both chronic and acute conditions—can now be controlled or cured. A wide range of patient advocacy groups, pressing for funding for AIDS, breast cancer, diabetes, and heart disease, seek public and private funds to continue the search for cures. From the March of Dimes to contemporary telethons, patient advocacy groups and the news media exhort the public to contribute to medical progress. Each year, new medical advances have underscored the narrative fidelity of this story, offering the public tangible proof of medicine's promise.

Proponents of this "no-crisis" view dismissed the notion that the nation was spending too much on health care. Critics charged the Clinton administration's Health Security Act threatened the pace of medical progress. "The $940 billion Americans spent on health care in 1993 did indeed represent a bit more than 14% of the nation's total output of goods and services. But by what standard is that too much? If we prefer to devote a larger proportion of our incomes to top quality health care than do other nations, what is wrong with that?" Narratives of progress described how additional spending fueled innovation, generating new treatments for individuals with chronic conditions such as asthma, allergies, depression, and erectile dysfunction. As a result, critics attacked the assumption that additional spending on health care was less productive than resources allocated to other purposes. As Charles Morris observes, "The social return from hip replacements that allow people to walk, ophthalmic surgery that restores sight, bypasses and stents that return people to work, and cancer screening must be as high as that from video games, VCRs, interactive porn, Arnold Schwarzenegger movies, 500-channel cable systems, jet skis, and behemoth four-wheel-drive cars." New medical advances continue to be regularly trumpeted by the media in "health beat" reports on local news and special reports on health published by leading newsmagazines and newspapers. News stories over the past decade echoed the same themes raised by their predecessors a quarter century earlier. The "main reason health care spending is rising is that modern medical technology has steadily made it possible to do more for more people. Hips and hearts can be fixed, while the ravages of schizophrenia and depression can be moderated."[30]

Despite continued concerns about the burden of health care costs, faith in the possibilities and promise of modern medicine has not faded. Writing in 2005, Senate majority leader William Frist (R-TN) captured the nation's continued faith in the power of medicine. As Frist noted, "There is plenty of evidence to suggest that these health care investments have paid handsome dividends. Life expectancy has increased from 47 to 77 years of age during the past 100 years. Hundreds of drugs are in the pipeline to treat conditions ranging from cancer to Alzheimer's disease." In contrast to crisis narratives that described the overuse of costly new diagnostic tools and pricey pharmaceuticals, Frist declared, "Rapidly advancing forms of technology are dramatically improving lives." By 2011 the director of the National Institutes of Health observed that medical research "is not a partisan issue. NIH's story is a compelling one of how modest investments have led to substantial improvements: longevity increasing about one year every six, disabilities reduced . . . all of these payoffs. The genome project from 1990 to 2003 spent about $4 billion to achieve a goal. What were the economic goods and services that came out of that? The Battelle study came up with $796 billion. So $796 billion to $4 billion, that's a 141 to 1 return on investment in 10 years."[31]

If health care spending is framed as an investment in longer life and better health rather than as waste, additional expenditures hardly constitute evidence of a growing crisis. In an affluent society, policy makers and the public may choose to spend more on health. From this vantage point, "it doesn't really matter what share of the GDP we spend on health care, just as it doesn't matter how much we spend on movies. We could spend 80 percent of GDP on movies and that would mean we were a wealthy society that liked to watch movies—and there's nothing ethically, morally, or economically wrong with that."[32] The decision to spend more on health care, in the end, reflects a value judgment, not a lack of policy tools. Stories of progress, therefore, undermine the notion of a "tipping point" where society spends too much on health care. In addition, if health care is viewed as an investment rather than a chronic problem to be "cured," reducing spending is a threat, not a solution.

As an issue, controlling health care costs at the societal level (as opposed to health insurance premiums or cost sharing) lacks traction with voters.

From 1973 to 1998, a majority of the public agreed that the nation was spending "too little" on health; by 1998 two out of three Americans favored additional spending "to improve and protect the nation's health." At no point did more than 9 percent of the public feel that the nation was spending "too much" on health. Indeed, polls conducted during the tumultuous debate over health care reform in 2009 found that while voters were worried about the cost of health care for themselves and their employers, they were less concerned about the nation's overall health care spending.[33]

For those who regard additional spending on health care as an investment, high health care costs simply reflect a "pronounced American cultural preference for medical progress." Public opinion polls consistently demonstrate a high level of support for medical research. Nearly all Americans (94 percent) regard medical research as important for the US economy, and more than half (55 percent) are willing to spend more to pay for it. Indeed, two-thirds of Americans (67 percent) were willing to pay an additional dollar per week in taxes to support additional medical research. As Robert Samuelson notes, "Americans receive more costly medical services than other people do, and pay more for them." The result, Samuelson asserts, is "a health care system that reflects our national values. It's highly individualistic, entrepreneurial, and suspicious of centralized supervision. Despite gripes about limits imposed by private insurers and Medicare, there are few effective controls on doctors and patients' choices. That's what most Americans want."[34]

Investments in basic research continue to enjoy bipartisan support. Indeed, "Congress has treated medical research as a favored child, with appropriations often exceeding the budget requests of the president. . . . When patients now complain about the escalating costs of care, they generally forget that many of the therapies available to them were unimaginable just a few years ago." Rising health care costs, in short, are an inadvertent, yet unavoidable, consequence of victory in the war against disease. "Spending more on health isn't necessarily bad. It isn't all rising prices, excessive drug makers' profits or unneeded care. Some reflects the growing American appetite for health care and costly life-improving advances in knowledge."[35]

Americans' support for investing in medical progress is evident in popular culture. In communities across the nation, millions of Americans join together in "walks for cures" to raise money for medical research and treatments, and tens of millions of Americans purchased LIVE STRONG bracelets or donned colored ribbons to express their support for continued progress in the war against disease. In particular, Lance Armstrong's successful battle

against cancer became a powerful symbol of the promise of medical progress. Pharmaceutical companies, for example, hailed Armstrong's triumph
over cancer as tangible proof of the payoff from pharmaceutical research
and development. As Food and Drug Administration commissioner Mark
McClellan argued in testimony before Congress in 2003, "Scientists and high
technology workers are making new discoveries and developing new products every day that are steadily improving the quality of our lives. This progress is critical to our health and our economic prosperity." Furthermore, a
Newsweek special report noted in 2005, "Scientific medicine has a special pull
on our imaginations. Like religion, it embraces our pain and our fears, and
assures us that things can be better. And for all its missteps, it often fulfills its
promise."[36] Celebrity survivors such as Lance Armstrong and Magic Johnson
featured prominently in popular newsmagazines and entertainment reports
as the faces of medical progress.

Pharmaceutical companies, medical device manufacturers, and other
opponents of government cost controls told their own stories of decline.
Efforts to control costs by setting prices for drugs were fraught with risk,
for "with lower prices, drug company profits will diminish and research and
development efforts may be reduced, resulting in a diminished flow of new
drugs." Ill-conceived cost-containment strategies threatened not only continued innovation, but also the lives, and quality of life, of millions of patients
and their families. "Good medicine itself may be at risk. Cut the drug payments and you cut drug research. Cut the hospital payments and the specialists will become hard to find. Cut the doctors enough, and there will be fewer
good doctors. If we want to continue with the high standard of medicine in
America, we may have to be willing to spend more."[37]

Health Care as Economic Progress

In addition, opponents of cost containment note that increased spending on
health care contributes to economic growth. Health care spending generates
income for a wide range of producers, including doctors, nurses, and hospitals in local communities around the nation. The health care industry has
been one of the fastest-growing areas of the US economy in recent decades.
By the late 1960s, news reports noted that "the boom in the health care field
has attracted many companies not related to medicine to plunge into the
healing industry up to their corporate clavicles." Far from being a crisis, additional spending on health care was a profitable business opportunity. "Many
companies have come to realize that the health care field is booming and

they want a piece of the action." Although talk of crisis dominated health policy debates in the late 1960s, the health care industry "captured the imagination of major American corporations—from General Electric to Litton Industries and Union Carbide to TRW. These and dozens more are actively developing new medical products or techniques."[38] Engineering and technology firms sought to address the industry's need for new systems to manage patient clinical and financial information, while scores of new medical device manufacturers sprouted up to meet the demand for new diagnostic and therapeutic tools.

The immense popularity of hospital construction, for example, led Congress to spread program funding throughout their districts, rather than funneling funds to poorer, rural areas. In 1969 news reports described the hospital industry as "a robust giant. . . . Today's 300,000 doctors, 650,000 nurses, and 2 million hospital workers will just about double in number in seven years." As a result, "in practically every community hospitals are adding personnel every day and paying sharply higher wages."[39] Far from being an unproductive backwater, businesses regarded health care as an engine of growth for the US economy.

At the local level, hospitals and nursing homes are often the largest employers in many communities. By the late 1980s, for example, the health care industry was the largest employer in the New York City economy. Health care outpaced banking, corporate headquarters, publishing, and real estate as a source of jobs. Writing in the *New England Journal of Medicine* in 1999, John Iglehart described the health care system as "a perpetual job creating enterprise."[40] In this context, additional spending on health care provides income and employment opportunities that are relatively immune to foreign competition. In the face of growing concerns over the outsourcing of jobs overseas, the health care industry retains an inherently local quality. In short, the very activities that critics view as wasteful spending provide jobs and income for millions of Americans who work in an industry that now represents one-seventh of the economy. In this context, calls for containing health care costs strike at the economic self-interest of millions of American families and businesses.

Opponents of cost control argued that government efforts to rein in spending had unintended side effects in an otherwise slack economy. The rate of job growth in the health sector exceeded the overall growth rate for the US economy in recent decades. By 2002 health care was the nation's largest industry, providing 12.9 million jobs in a wide range of settings, from

highly trained professionals such as physicians to clerical workers and support staff for hospitals, nursing homes, and medical offices. Current employment forecasts suggest that the demand for health care services will continue to expand in the coming decades. Ten of the nation's fastest-growing
occupations are now in the health care field; between 2002 and 2012, health
care was projected to add more jobs than any other industry in the United
States.[41]

Fears of Rationing

Opponents of cost containment also warned of the dangerous consequences
of adopting "painful prescriptions" such as rationing health care. Providers
portrayed proposals to limit access to beneficial, and perhaps lifesaving, services presently covered by private health insurance plans as a slippery slope.
During each debate over cost controls from the 1970s to 2010, the medical
profession stoked opposition to cost containment by warning that patients
would be unable to obtain needed care. Hospital administrators defended
the rising cost of care in the 1970s, noting that "we apply the fruits of progress in medical science and technology without stint to the many, and bring
massive resources to bear in salvaging a single individual. Who would have
us do otherwise?" In 1979 legislators opposed to the Carter administration's
proposed bill to contain hospital costs argued that spending more on health
was the right thing to do, because "the American people demand the best."
Opponents of cost controls employed stories of decline that described the
painful consequences of rationing for patients and their families. As Representative Phil Gramm (R-TX) cautioned in 1979, "Babies in Alabama and
Texas are going to die" if Congress denied smaller rural hospitals the opportunity to acquire the latest medical technologies. By the early 1980s, physicians argued that the cure for rising costs could be worse than the disease.
As the president of the AMA noted in 1981, "When you start manipulating a
system that treats three million people a day you'd better be a little careful
before jumping off the cliff."[42]

Similar warnings about the consequences of rationing galvanized opposition to health care reform during the Clinton administration. Opponents
mocked Democratic proposals for health care reform, asking, "Should we
destroy the world's finest medical care, in hopes of helping to rescue the irresponsible?" Writing in the *New York Times*, William Safire charged that the
administration's proposed price controls "(euphemized as 'premium caps')
require rationing, or denial—and most of us do not want the health care we

already have taken away." In her widely cited article in the *New Republic,* conservative commentator Elizabeth McCaughey argued, "If you are seriously ill, the best place to be is in the United States. Among all industrialized nations, the United States has the highest cure rates for stomach, cervical, and uterine cancers, the second highest cure rate for breast cancer, and is second to none in treating heart disease." This assessment reinforced notions of American exceptionalism that celebrated investments in health care as a responsible choice. From this vantage point, government cost controls threatened not only access to medical treatments for patients, but also American technological prowess and leadership in medical innovation. The Heritage Foundation charged that the Clinton plan "would set up a new National Health Board to tell us what medical services we can and cannot have, how much money we are allowed to spend on health care each year and how many physicians will be trained to serve us and in what specialties."[43] Images of depersonalized "assembly line" clinics and long waits for specialists and surgical procedures evoked concerns about the erosion of high-quality care as an unintended side effect of cost containment.

Similar fears of rationing resurfaced in the summer of 2009, as members of Congress held town hall meetings with constituents over proposed health care reforms. "Although administration officials are eager to deny it," Martin Feldstein argued, "rationing health care is central to President Barack Obama's health plan. The Obama strategy is to reduce health costs by rationing the services that we and future generations of patients will receive." Fears that price controls and government-led "death panels" would ration care generated visceral opposition to the Obama administration's efforts to win support for health care reform. As Senator Tom Coburn (R-OK) warned senior citizens during a heated exchange over proposed cuts in Medicare payments, "I have a message for you. You're going to die sooner." Republican attacks on Democratic reform proposals echoed the objections leveled against the Clinton health plan fifteen years earlier. As Representative John Boehner (R-OH), the ranking Republican in the House of Representatives, wrote, "The president claimed that the plan will not lead to rationing. But the bill . . . would create a 'Health Benefits Advisory Committee' that would make determinations about what kinds of treatments, items and services can be covered."[44] Boehner's warning paralleled Elizabeth McCaughey's attack on the Clinton Health Security Act in 1993, for it raised the specter of government officials tightening health benefits over time to control costs.

Conclusion

Despite decades of debate, health care costs continue to surge. In 2011 health care accounted for more than 17 percent of the US GDP, and per capita health expenditures rose from $143 in 1960 to $4,670 in 2000. Estimates of future health care spending are sobering. As the *Wall Street Journal* editorialized in 2009, "Every public or private attempt to arrest this climb [in health care costs] has failed; wage and price controls in the 1970s; the insurance industry's 'voluntary effort' in the '80s; managed care in the '90s." The chronic nature of health care inflation compounds the challenge of cost. Health care costs represent "a slow and steady decline, producing no crisis, no Pearl Harbor, no 9/11. As a result we seem incapable of grappling with it seriously." Year after year, costs rise—and the increase in health care costs routinely exceeds the overall rate of inflation in the economy. Language lies at the root of our cost-containment conundrum, for as Daniel Callahan notes, "Cost controls that are likely to be politically acceptable will not be very effective, and what might be effective will not be acceptable."[45]

To date, reformers have embraced the language of crisis in an effort to arouse an apathetic and quiescent public. Political candidates and policy analysts have focused their attention on *how* to control costs, treating the need for cost control as a foregone conclusion. It is not. The crux of the problem facing reformers is that there is no real constituency for cost control within the American public. Dire warnings of impending collapse and economic catastrophe lack narrative fidelity, for each year the health care system continues to provide quality care to most Americans. Since past predictions of collapse failed to materialize, future warnings that "the sky is falling" with respect to health care costs face an increasingly skeptical public, despite ongoing concerns about rising insurance premiums. As a result, reformers must build a case for cost containment rather than treat it as an axiom in policy debates.

The duality of health care spending makes the existence of a cost crisis in health care a matter of perspective. Patients and purchasers of care decry rising expenditures, but these costs represent income for providers, a source of economic growth for many communities, and hope for patients and families struggling with illness. Health providers tend to view their own products and services as necessary, while questioning "waste" elsewhere in the system. Despite decades of crisis rhetoric, consumers continue to press for more coverage and additional services, not less.

The public's unwillingness to confront the difficult trade-offs in cost containment is not new. Indeed, public confusion over health care spending has characterized each debate over health care reform. As early as 1968, health economist Victor Fuchs noted that the "weighing of costs against benefits can be found almost everywhere in the economy, but when we come to health, there is a deep seated reluctance to do it." More than two decades later, David Mechanic observed that "while most people agree, in principle, that excess hospital beds should be converted or eliminated, in practice they want the principle to apply only to other people's hospitals." The public remains conflicted about health care costs, for while the rising cost of health care is a leading concern, more than half of Americans also believe the United States should increase its commitment to health-related research. Furthermore, the constituencies targeted by reformers, the "health care industry and its workers, business, labor, and various consumer groups . . . [are] convinced that cost control should begin somewhere else."[46] The rhetorical shortcomings of crisis narratives reflect this tension; for much of the public, the relevant policy question is not how best to control costs, but whether doing so is necessary or desirable in the first place. In this context, narratives that presume the existence of a crisis are doomed to fail, for the pursuit of cost containment remains a perilous proposition for policy makers.

To paraphrase British writer G. K. Chesterton's description of Christianity, cost containment has not been tried and found wanting in America; it has been found difficult and not tried.[47] Reformers who seek to "bend the curve" of health care spending in the United States need to focus less attention on the specifics of policy proposals and more time on how to explain the need for controlling costs to average Americans. Rising costs cannot be cured but must be managed. Doing so requires a rhetorical shift by reformers, for opponents of reform have always offered powerful rebuttals to the rhetoric of crisis. Policy makers and issue entrepreneurs must connect cost containment to deep-seated, widely shared values such as efficiency that resonate with the public that also reflect the notion of health care as an investment. Successful strategies for cost containment must acknowledge the public's desire for medical progress. Leadership to build support for containing health care costs, therefore, must begin with a discussion of the value of health services provided to the public, laying a foundation for a national conversation about where additional spending will do the most good.

CHAPTER THREE

The Medical Malpractice Crisis

Doctors want to reduce the rights of victims. It's like saying the way to solve muggings is to change the penal law so that mugging is not a crime. That's not the solution. The root of the problem is sloppy medical care.
> —New York State Trial Lawyers Association, quoted in Tom Goldstein,
> "Doctors Called Opposed to Rights," *New York Times,* June 3, 1975

For the past several years, we have seen numerous symptoms that tell us our nation is facing a crisis because of a broken medical liability system. The symptoms are unmistakable: patients having to leave their state to receive urgent surgical care; pregnant women who cannot find an obstetrician to monitor their pregnancy and deliver their babies; community health centers reducing their services or closing their doors because of liability insurance concerns and the increasing fear of litigation; efforts to improve patient safety and quality being stifled because of lawsuit fears.
> —American Medical Association, "Testimony Before the Committee on
> Energy and Commerce, Subcommittee on Health,
> U.S. House of Representatives," February 10, 2005

DEBATES OVER MALPRACTICE REFORM in the United States evoke a strong sense of déjà vu. The same themes used to frame the debate over the malpractice crisis in the 1970s—including familiar policy narratives, horror stories, and recurring patterns of news coverage and political rhetoric—reappeared in each subsequent debate about malpractice reform. The rhetorical similarities are so striking, in fact, that legislative testimony, editorials, and news coverage from the 1970s or mid-1980s could easily be mistaken for rhetoric from the present day, and vice versa. For decades, physicians defined the malpractice crisis as an insurance crisis, typified by out-of-control growth in claims, the size of jury awards, and malpractice insurance premiums. Lawyers, in contrast, argued that physicians were the real culprits behind the malpractice crisis, as the profession was either unwilling or incapable of preventing "bad doctors" from committing serious, often deadly, medical errors. Both diagnoses, however, are ultimately incomplete.[1]

The debate over malpractice reform over the past four decades illustrates Wittgenstein's discussion of the "unintended misuse" of language. Rather than engaging in a serious dialogue about how to reduce the rate of malpractice and preventable medical errors, the principal characters in each narrative—doctors and lawyers—continue to talk past each other, recycling familiar arguments each time the issue returns to the public agenda. Despite decades of debate and the passage of scores of malpractice reforms, no agreement exists on either the nature of the crisis or how to treat it. Neither diagnosis, however, addresses the underlying problem of unintended medical errors that claim tens of thousands of lives in America each year. As a result, talk of a malpractice crisis is ultimately dysfunctional, for it fails to focus public attention on efforts to improve the safety and reliability of medical care.

For physicians, the rhetoric of crisis became a powerful symbol to mobilize support for tort reforms among legislators and the public. Medical malpractice cases are tort claims, in which an individual alleges that he or she has been injured as a result of the negligence of another party. Although tort reforms offered short-term relief for rising malpractice premiums, they did little to address the underlying problem of medical error. Little evidence exists that tort reforms reduce the cost of "defensive medicine," in which doctors order additional tests and treatments to shield themselves from charges of medical practice. Physicians framed each malpractice crisis from the 1970s to the present day as an insurance crisis, but failed to acknowledge the widespread prevalence of preventable medical error. Furthermore, while the number of malpractice claims, and the average size of jury awards, increased over time, they have done so at a steady, incremental pace. Spikes in the number of claims, in other words, do not seem to explain rising premiums for physicians. Dire predictions that rising malpractice premiums would lead to physician shortages also failed to materialize.

The policy narratives offered by opponents of tort reform suffer from similar shortcomings. The legal profession focused public attention on the victims of egregious errors. Trial lawyers, for their part, generalized from "worst cases" to raise doubts about the competence of the medical profession and the safety of patients. Most Americans, however, continued to receive high-quality health care without suffering grievous injuries at the hands of negligent providers. As early as 1971, observers noted that "as a means of improving the quality of medical care," the malpractice system was "capricious, extravagant, and works only after the fact." The threat of malpractice is designed to deter physicians from providing substandard care, but most injured patients do not sue (and, indeed, are often not aware that an error occurred). As a result, most doctors who commit medical errors are not held accountable in court, and most injured patients receive no compensation. In addition, many cases where patients did receive compensation, through either a settlement or a jury verdict, showed no evidence of clinical negligence on the part of physicians (for example, failing to follow the standard of care).[2] Thus, both supporters and opponents of malpractice reform rely upon incomplete, if not inaccurate, diagnoses to structure public deliberation over how to address the system's shortcomings.

The rhetoric of malpractice reform has an ironic twist, for the misperceptions, myths, and stereotypes that dominate public discussions of medical malpractice undermine the prospects for collaboration needed to reduce the incidence of preventable medical errors. Crisis talk also encouraged policy makers to pursue short-term solutions designed to limit the growth of premiums, rather than long-term efforts to improve patient safety and decrease the incidence of claims. Crises are not conducive to a deliberative approach to policy problems. Demands by doctors and insurers for immediate relief from legislators swept away the complexities and nuances of the issue, leading lawmakers to focus on tort reform as a popular "quick fix." State tort reforms, however, have not reduced the number of lawsuits. As an organizing principle, crisis offers a particularly poor description of the problems plaguing state insurance markets. During each "crisis," most doctors continued to see patients despite the higher cost of doing so. Malpractice insurance premiums also followed a cyclical pattern over the past four decades despite repeated efforts to fix the system's shortcomings.[3] Upon closer inspection, premium increases are a chronic, recurring problem for malpractice insurance markets rather than an acute condition. As a result, recurring talk of a malpractice insurance crisis hinders, rather than helps, efforts to reduce the prevalence and incidence of medical malpractice itself.

Narratives of Crisis

Public discourse about medical malpractice reform has evolved little since 1975, when the president of the American Medical Association appeared at the annual meeting of the American Bar Association. Urging doctors and lawyers to work together in search of solutions, he noted that "some physicians have said publicly that greedy lawyers are the major cause of medical professional liability problems and that the contingent fee is the primary factor in the high cost of litigation. And some attorneys—particularly trial lawyers engaged in medical professional liability problems—would have the public believe that the proximate cause of the malpractice insurance crisis is the near total incompetency of a major portion of the medical profession."[4] Debates about malpractice reform are characterized by disjunction between the rhetoric of crisis and the lived experiences of patients and providers.

Fear has short-circuited debate over malpractice reform for decades. Fear-based appeals for malpractice reform infused policy debates with a strong sense of urgency. As the president of the American Medical Association declared in 1975, "The malpractice problem is so critical that if the legislatures do not respond to remedial legislation we are absolutely going to have utter chaos in this country because for the first time in history you are going to see massive walkouts and withholding of services by American doctors."[5] Images of physicians closing their practices, leaving desperate patients scrambling for treatment, played upon the latent fears of patients and their families that lifesaving care would not be available when it was most needed. Even though most doctors continued to treat patients during each "crisis" period, walkouts and warnings of an emerging shortage of physicians resonated with the public because of the intensely personal nature of the doctor-patient relationship. Malpractice debates underscored the multiple meanings embedded in crisis rhetoric: while the public remained sympathetic to the plight of injured patients, significant increases in the cost of malpractice insurance raised fears that care would not be available when it was most needed.

Physicians often conveyed the need for tort reform using familiar terminology from popular television medical dramas. In 2002, for example, the president of the West Virginia Medical Association described the exodus of providers as a "code blue" situation and warned that "practically every day, doctors are leaving." A year later, Pennsylvania physicians adopted similar language, describing their public rally for malpractice reform as a "Code Blue" emergency protest.[6] The use of such medical terminology—often familiar to the public from popular television programs—underscored the notion that the system was fast approaching a breaking point.

Physicians and other supporters of reform framed the debate over rising premiums using stories of decline. By 1985 the American Medical Association warned that medical malpractice costs had again reached "crisis proportions." When physicians faced triple-digit increases in malpractice rates in 2003, the AMA declared that eighteen states faced a new malpractice crisis. President George W. Bush invoked the same policy narrative that framed debates over reform in the 1970s, arguing that "we must confront the frivo-lous lawsuits that are driving up the cost of health care and hurting doctors and patients."[7] This is a powerful narrative that fosters political mobilization, for its characters (for example, doctors) are both familiar and well liked.

The stories used to frame public discourse about malpractice reform also displayed a remarkable consistency over time. Television and print news reports accentuated the nationwide reach of the developing crisis. Media coverage emphasized the scope and proximity of the issue for average Amer-icans, even those who lived in states not yet affected by the crisis. As *ABC News* reported in 1987, "The American Medical Association is warning that the problems in Florida are not unique and the crisis that has occurred here could easily occur elsewhere." Indeed, spokesmen for the medical profession often noted the danger of the crisis spreading to other states. Nearly two decades later, the *Saturday Evening Post* informed readers that "a crisis [is] putting American lives at risk. . . . It occurs when a pregnant woman is in labor—and no obstetrician is available. Or when a nine-year-old boy has a head injury, but there's no neurosurgeon remaining in his area. Or when a town's only trauma center shuts down for want of physicians."[8] Even though most patients did not experience disruptions of care, stories of doctors forced to close their practices or curtail services reinforced the proximity of the issue for patients. Such dire, albeit vague, warnings raised an implicit question for the public: will my hospital, or my doctor, be next? In this narra-tive, rising rates affect all Americans.

Both the mass media and policy makers defined trial lawyers as a sym-bolic enemy during each debate over medical malpractice reform. Demo-crats and Republicans, incumbents and challengers, railed against the pro-liferation of "jackpot justice." In 2004, for example, President George W. Bush argued that "in order to make sure we've got good docs practicing medicine, to make sure health care is affordable, we need to stop these junk lawsuits." His opponent, Senator John Kerry (D-MA), concurred, noting that "one of the things I intend to do is to do a better job of holding down medical malprac-tice costs." Kerry declared, "We need a national system in place that will weed out the irresponsible lawsuits without taking away patients' rights." Demo-crats, however, remained decidedly less enthusiastic about tort reform than their Republican colleagues. Speaking before the American Medical Associa-tion in 2009, President Barack Obama pledged to "work with the AMA so we can scale back the excessive defensive medicine that reinforces our current system, and shift to a system where we are providing better care."[9] Obama, however, refused to endorse caps on malpractice awards supported by physicians, congressional Republicans, and many governors.

The First Diagnosis: A Liability Crisis

Concerns about spiraling malpractice premiums attracted widespread attention in the early 1970s, as many private malpractice insurers withdrew from some markets and stopped writing new policies in others. The language used by policy makers over the past four decades underscored the need to confront an emerging crisis. The Nixon administration's Commission on Medical Malpractice compared the crisis to "a proliferation of cancerous cells which have spread throughout the health care system." By late 1974, the US Department of Health, Education, and Welfare (HEW) warned that "physicians in at least seven states face the prospect of not being able to obtain insurance when their present policies expire." Within months, several of the nation's largest medical malpractice insurers declared bankruptcy or refused to renew their existing policies. By April 1975 the *New York Times* editorialized that the "malpractice crisis . . . has assumed national proportions. In many states physicians and hospitals now face the possibility that within the next few months they may have no malpractice insurance at all, or will be able to buy it only on terms that will put it beyond reach."[10]

Medical malpractice first attracted widespread attention during the mid-nineteenth century. The rate of malpractice suits increased dramatically as physicians developed new procedures and formalized professional standards of practice. New techniques and therapies offered benefits to patients, but also afforded new grounds for litigation. This burst of litigation led to a "deep chasm" between physicians and lawyers that persisted over time. By the middle of the twentieth century, the growing number of malpractice claims led the *Journal of the American Medical Association* to warn doctors that "professional liability must be considered as an occupational hazard for every physician."[11] Although malpractice reform sparked widespread interest at both the state and national levels, neither policy makers nor the public defined the issue as a crisis.

Before the 1970s, relatively few physicians were sued for malpractice, as prevailing legal standards shielded most physicians from claims of medical negligence. Under the "locality rule," for example, the testimony of nationally recognized experts was not admissible in most state courts; providers' actions were compared to the standard of care in the community. In this environment, most medical malpractice cases were decided in favor of the defendants, and malpractice insurance premiums remained relatively low. In the early 1950s, for example, premiums for a typical malpractice policy in New York ranged from $64 per year in upstate counties to $106 in the New York City metropolitan area. As changes in legal procedures made it easier for patients to win negligence claims against physicians, however, malpractice filings soared. The number of lawsuits filed against physicians increased more than tenfold over four decades, from 1.3 per 100 physicians in 1960 to 15 per 100 physicians in 2003. As Richard Anderson noted in 2004, although the frequency of medical malpractice claims has changed little in recent years, 1 out of 6 physicians reports a claim each year. "On any given day, there are more than 120,000 malpractice actions pending against physicians."[12] As the number of lawsuits increased, malpractice insurers passed along the cost to physicians in the form of higher premiums.

Media reports in the early 1970s highlighted the plight of physicians whose insurance premiums increased several fold. The emerging crisis reached a national television audience in 1975 when doctors in Mansfield, Ohio, refused to perform elective surgeries after their malpractice insurer carriers refused to renew their coverage. News coverage of the issue focused on the implications for patients and their families and framed the malpractice crisis in terms of decreased access to care. In protest, doctors refused to perform surgeries; anesthesiologists interviewed by the *CBS Evening News* urged Ohio legislators to take prompt action to control spiraling premiums.[13]

The emerging crisis reached a boiling point in California in the spring of 1975, as anesthesiologists and surgeons throughout the San Francisco Bay Area refused to perform elective procedures to protest proposed premium hikes. On May 1—when the doctors' strike began—the crisis was featured on all three network news broadcasts. Both *NBC* and *ABC* dedicated more than 10 percent of their evening news broadcasts to the issue. Television audiences learned about the crisis through powerful visual images of doctors clad in white lab coats marching on the California Legislature. Striking physicians warned viewers that without significant reforms, they could no longer afford to continue practicing medicine. The walkout—which included more than two thousand physicians in northern California—lasted for twenty-eight days. By the second week of May, physicians in Los Angeles and San Diego also staged protests against rising rates.[14]

Fear was a common theme in network news coverage of the California walkout. For nearly a month, news broadcasts featured interviews with physicians threatening to close or relocate their practices. News reports profiled desperate hospital administrators who wondered how long their institutions might be able to "hold on" without performing elective surgeries. During the strike, hospitals in northern California canceled scheduled surgeries and laid off more than thirteen thousand workers, and some hospitals threatened to close their doors unless legislators found a solution to doctors' malpractice woes. Horror stories focused attention on the plight of individual physicians struggling to pay rising premiums and underscored the need for urgent action. For example, *NBC Nightly News* described the plight of a rural doctor who planned to relocate to Wyoming after his annual malpractice premiums increased 360 percent. Reporters warned audiences that without immediate action, patients could be left in a state of medical limbo waiting for surgery.[15]

Striking doctors in California offered a now familiar diagnosis of the emerging malpractice crisis. Physicians blamed spiraling medical malpractice premiums on a rash of frivolous lawsuits filed by overzealous attorneys and litigious patients. Without reforms to limit both the number and the size of malpractice lawsuits, physicians warned that "we will all be faced with the absolute impossibility of practicing." The physician walkout prompted the California Medical Association to convene an emergency meeting for the first time since the raucous debate over "socialized medicine" in the late 1940s. The CMA's president endorsed the work stoppage, arguing that "a physician, in good conscience, may deem it necessary to delay elective medical and surgical procedures or to absent himself temporarily from his office to focus the attention of the public, the Legislature, and the Governor on this crisis."[16]

In the wake of the California walkout, talk of an emerging malpractice crisis soon appeared in other states. Doctors in Florida, New York, Pennsylvania, and Texas followed the lead of their colleagues in California. In the spring of 1975, delegates at the New York Medical Society's annual convention resolved that the "rights of our patients to have their medical needs met is presently in jeopardy. The House of Delegates is convinced that the rights of our patients now rest in the hands of our elected representative in Albany and only through the passage of meaningful legislation will these rights be preserved."[17]

In California the crisis subsided after legislators enacted a landmark tort reform bill—the Medical Injury Compensation Reform Act—in the months following the strike. This legislation, which imposed a $250,000 cap on noneconomic damages for "pain and suffering," soon became a model for malpractice reforms in other states. By 1980 most states had followed California's lead by enacting tort reforms such as pretrial review panels, joint underwriting associations, and limits on malpractice awards designed to limit the number of malpractice cases and the size of malpractice verdicts. Doctors also formed their own insurance companies—dubbed "bedpan mutuals"—in the wake of the malpractice crisis in the 1970s, but these physician-owned insurers soon experienced the same financial problems as traditional insurers.

The same tactics employed by doctors during the medical malpractice crisis of 1975—from physician strikes to public rallies by doctors clad in scrubs and lab coats—reappeared again from the mid-1980s to the present. Doctors' tactics were designed to both break legislative logjams and preempt alternative definitions of the medical malpractice crisis. The power of this symbolic strategy is evident in its persistence over time, as protests reappeared across the nation during each crisis period. In 2002, for example, doctors in Florida held public rallies to warn policy makers of a new "medical emergency" created by skyrocketing malpractice costs. In January 2003, *NBC Nightly News* warned viewers once again that "doctors [are] going on strike. The surgeons in West Virginia are calling this a walkout to protest the ever higher price of buying medical malpractice insurance, which in turn reflects the ever higher awards in medical malpractice cases. Call it what you will—a walkout or a strike—it is a health care crisis spreading across this country." Later that year, *ABC News* reported that "doctors in West Palm Beach walked off the job, warning that high premiums are forcing them out of their practices." An estimated 70 percent of physicians in New Jersey also embraced this familiar protest strategy in 2003, as physicians closed their offices, postponed nonemergency surgeries, and marched to the state capitol.[18] By withdrawing doctors' services, physician strikes heightened public anxiety and concern.

Following the lead of California physicians in the 1970s, doctors took to the streets during each successive malpractice crisis to make "house calls" on legislators. Images of striking physicians dramatized the seriousness of the crisis and stoked public fears about the continued availability of medical care. In 1985 viewers watching ABC's coverage of a physician walkout in Michigan, for example, learned that "so many doctors were here, more than 9,000, that virtually all non-emergency surgery across the state was canceled." News coverage over the next two decades evoked a strong sense of déjà vu. In 2003 *Good Morning America* reported that 20 percent of doctors in Pennsylvania were "now out in the streets and saying something must be changed." That same year, *CBS Evening News* noted that "around the country, physicians are putting down their stethoscopes and picking up picket signs, calling for legislation to limit jury awards to hold down medical malpractice premiums."[19]

The positive image of the medical profession shielded physicians from a public backlash as doctors canceled appointments and rescheduled surgeries to lobby legislators and march to state capitols. During the debate over tort reform in the US Senate in 1995, for example, "the tenor of the debate underscored that elected officials afford doctors far more respect than they do lawyers. Several senators . . . lashed out at trial lawyers, depicting them as obstacles to such change who are trying to make money on people's misery." However, "even those senators who opposed the doctors always spoke respectfully of the medical profession."[20] Although doctors' actions often disrupted care for their own patients, physicians enjoyed continued support from policy makers and the public as they sought relief from rising rates.

Several distinct but complementary themes define reformers' narratives of a medical liability crisis. First, physicians argued that out-of-control premiums were an *unaffordable* burden. Second, physicians warned that without dramatic action, lifesaving care would be *unavailable,* as doctors retired or relocated in response to rising premiums in "crisis" states. Policy makers and providers also charged that defensive medicine—the additional tests and procedures ordered by doctors to protect themselves from potential lawsuits—contributed to *uncontrollable* health care spending. Reformers offered several stories of control to resolve the crisis, including proposals to cap the size of jury awards for "pain and suffering" and limit the number of malpractice suits.

The medical profession made the financial burden of insurance coverage a central theme in each crisis period. As early as 1971, physicians complained that "premiums in some areas have gone up tenfold in a decade." From 1960 to 1972, the average cost of malpractice premiums for "low-risk" physicians increased almost 600 percent, while physicians in "high-risk" categories faced increases of about 900 percent. By the mid-1980s, physicians in New York spent roughly 10 percent of their gross income on medical malpractice insurance. In 1974, HEW secretary Caspar Weinberger labeled rising insurance costs for physicians as a crisis, warning that "physicians in at least seven states face the prospect of not being able to obtain insurance when their present policies expire." The following year, the president of the AMA described malpractice as "the number one problem that faces the American medical profession." This sentiment was echoed by both state legislators and members of Congress in the mid-1970s. Speaking before the US House of Representatives in 1975, Representative James F. Hastings (R-NY) declared that "the availability and cost of medical malpractice insurance has reached emergency proportions in many states because of dramatically increased claims and skyrocketing award levels."[21] In subsequent years, Hastings's warning was repeated by scores of policy makers, medical societies, and other supporters of tort reform.

Three decades after Weinberger's warning, advocates of reform once again evoked the rhetoric of crisis, using similar images and examples to dramatize the need for swift action. Writing in the *New England Journal of Medicine* in 2003, Michelle Mello, David Studdart, and Troyen Brennan repeated the same policy narrative that defined previous malpractice debates in the 1970s:

> A major medical malpractice crisis is unfolding in the United States today. The American Medical Association has identified 18 states in which physicians and institutional health care providers are having grave difficulties obtaining affordable professional liability insurance. In the past two years, insurance premiums in those states have increased dramatically for physicians in high-risk specialties such as obstetrics, emergency medicine, general surgery, surgical sub-specialties, and radiology. Another 26 states are on "orange alert" with indicators suggesting a serious and worsening situation. Physicians in West Virginia, New Jersey, Florida, Pennsylvania, Mississippi, Illinois, Texas, and Missouri have held or threatened work stoppages to draw attention to their plight, and several hospitals in the states that have been hit the hardest have temporarily closed or threatened to close emergency room [ER], obstetrical, or other services.[22]

Such warnings underscored the national scope of rising malpractice rates, bolstering the case for swift action. In addition, the threat of service disruptions, affecting the ability of patients to obtain care from their doctors, was defined as a growing problem.

Doctors also cited the financial burden of rising malpractice premiums as evidence of a worsening crisis. As the nation celebrated its bicentennial in 1976, the American Surgical Association complained that "the insurance premiums for a single year are, in some cases, more than the doctor could hope to earn in his first year of practice." Physicians argued that spiraling malpractice rates would dissuade doctors from practicing in high-cost states and would encourage promising young doctors to consider less risky areas of medical practice. A decade later, policy makers continued to repeat the same call to arms. Senator Dan Quayle (R-IN) expressed outrage that "insurers are now asking for premiums rate increases in excess of 100 percent a year" even as the overall rate of inflation moderated.[23]

A rapid increase in malpractice premiums also produced a similar outcry within the medical profession in the past decade. As Philip Howard argued in 2002, "American justice has created a crisis in American health care. . . . American justice is causing health care to suffer a kind of nervous break-down." This view was echoed by President George W. Bush, who declared, "Some insurers are now dropping medical liability coverage for doctors. . . . Higher and higher insurance premiums make it nearly impossible for a lot of doctors to practice medicine, and if docs don't practice medicine, it's hard to have good health care. Without insurance, they cannot afford to treat patients." *CBS News* also reinforced the notion of an affordability crisis in 2003, informing viewers, "Doctors argue that they're going out of business because of the exploding cost of malpractice insurance." As *ABC News* reported in 2002, "For many doctors in high risk fields, insurance is now unaffordable." A similar story appeared in 2004, as *CBS News* informed viewers that "across the country, doctors say rising insurance costs are driving them out of business."[24]

Horror stories of the financial burdens of malpractice coverage abound. Appeals for tort reform often use extreme cases to personalize the impact of rising malpractice rates on individual physicians and their patients. In 2002 President Bush cited the example of a Nevada physician who chose to leave the state after his malpractice premiums rose from $33,000 per year to $108,000, even though he himself had never been sued. The president argued that "the trial lawyers, suit after suit after suit, have driven this good man out of Nevada." Television news coverage of malpractice reinforced this story of financial ruin. Heart-wrenching news segments described the plight of physicians driven from practice by escalating costs. By 1985 *ABC News* reported that "half of Michigan's obstetricians have quit, unable to afford liability coverage." *ABC News* introduced viewers to Dr. Daniel O'Keefe, a veteran obstetrician who delivered nearly ten thousand babies over three decades of practice in rural New York, who had decided to close his practice because "the cost of insuring himself against future lawsuits had grown too high." The reporter noted that "the trauma for doctors comes from a 300% increase since 1975 in malpractice claims nationwide." In a similar profile, *ABC News* interviewed another obstetrician from Michigan who had also been delivering babies for twenty-five years whose malpractice premiums increased 300 percent. The doctor warned that "if the trend continues, we may not be here a year from now practicing obstetrics. . . . [We'll be] [o]ut of business."[25] Similar stories of doctors forced to retire or relocate their practices reappeared in each "crisis" period.

Spectacular jury awards also featured prominently in the stories of decline told by reformers. Doctors and insurers cited the rapid growth in the size of malpractice jury awards in their calls for malpractice reform. Mammoth verdicts became commonplace. The average payment per claim, including jury awards and out-of-court settlements, increased more than 12 percent per year for physicians and 19 percent for hospitals between 1971 and 1978. In 1983, for example, a Brooklyn jury awarded a five-year-old girl more than $29 million. Two decades later, another New York jury awarded $140 million to a child who suffered permanent brain damage after surgery. In the wake of this decision, insurers warned that "medical malpractice premium costs will at least double, and in some cases, I think the insurers just won't write coverage at all."[26] Although most malpractice cases were decided in favor of defendants, the scale of jury awards to plaintiffs continued to rise.

A complementary story of decline described the impact of rising malpractice rates on the availability of health care services. Fear also featured prominently in this policy narrative. A. O. Hirschman describes the threat of exit as a powerful rhetorical tool in *Exit, Voice, and Loyalty.* Physicians argued that rising rates would make care unavailable for patients, as the high cost of malpractice in "crisis" states drove doctors to retire or relocate.

During the 1975 strike by California physicians, a wide range of news reports profiled doctors who threatened to either quit the profession or relocate their practices because of rising malpractice costs. These same concerns surfaced again a decade later. As the *New York Times* editorialized in 1985, "Doctors' liability is more than a personal concern. Those who can't get full coverage have begun to reject patients. The huge premiums discourage young doctors from establishing practices and make it harder to provide good medical care in poor neighborhoods." Television news coverage also played upon public anxieties of an impending doctor shortage, presenting vivid profiles of visible victims to viewers. By 1987 *ABC News* reported that the "soaring cost of medical malpractice insurance has now reached crisis proportions in southern Florida. Doctors have been refusing to staff emergency rooms." News reports described sick or injured patients unable to receive emergency care and physicians who could not afford, or in some cases even obtain, malpractice coverage. *ABC News* warned, "If you need emergency care in southern Florida's Dade County you may be in trouble. Up to 22 hospitals have substantially limited their emergency facilities and for critically injured patients there are only two trauma centers operating in the area. The cutback was brought on by the staggering cost of medical malpractice insurance. A new state law forces some physicians who service emergency rooms to carry insurance they say they simply cannot afford."[27]

News reports in the late 1980s described southern Florida as "medicine's Beirut. Though rescue squads are not digging through rubble, they are trying to cope with assisting victims in counties where most hospital emergency rooms have stopped accepting trauma patients." This analogy was jarring, for television coverage of the civil war in Lebanon in the early 1980s was defined by graphic images of violence and disorder. Describing the health care system in one of the nation's largest and most populous cities in these terms suggested that the health care system itself was on the brink of collapse. This story of decline emphasized the proximity of malpractice reform for average Americans, regardless of where they lived. As one medical society president noted in 1988, "We are in the midst of a liability crisis in Florida that threatens the quality of life of every one of us."[28] In this narrative, rising malpractice rates not only were a problem for physicians, but impacted all of society—both the healthy and the sick—who might need a doctor.

The same story of decline reappeared again in subsequent decades. In 2003 the president of the Florida Medical Association declared, "We're approaching Third World medicine where people are traveling 100 miles to get specialized care." This same story appeared in debates over malpractice reform around the nation. Viewers of the *CBS News Early Show* learned that "if you need an operation and you're in West Virginia that might not be the place to be this morning . . . because more than two dozen surgeons at four hospitals [are] on their second day of a walkout protesting the high cost of malpractice insurance." The litany of hospital closures and physician departures reinforced the severity and scope of the crisis for television audiences. The president-elect of the American Medical Association predicted grave consequences for the medical profession unless steps were taken to address the malpractice crisis. "Not only are people deciding not to go into ob-gyn, they're deciding not to go into medicine. The whole profession is at risk." The result, as *NBC Nightly News* anchor Tom Brokaw warned viewers in 2004, is "a kind of medical migration, sending doctors away from their longtime patients, breaking still another traditional bond in American health care."[29]

Warnings about a crisis of access portrayed the medical malpractice crisis as a national, not a regional, concern. By the 1980s, news reports emphasized the broadening scope of the crisis, underscoring the proximity of the issue for audiences. "Faced with a growing number of malpractice claims and the rising expectations of patients," reporters informed the public that "a significant number of the nation's doctors have either abandoned the practice of obstetrics or are seriously considering it." As Senator Orrin Hatch (R-UT) noted in 1990, "Physicians' concerns over future liability costs is adversely affecting access to care for all of us." A decade later, officials from the West Virginia Medical Association described the medical malpractice crisis as "a life-and-death issue for patients in West Virginia in the ability to get access to care." By 2002 *Time* warned readers that "millions across America might turn up for an appointment one day soon and find that the doctor is out—for good. Thousands have already lost their doctors to a malpractice crisis that, while concentrated for now in certain states and specialties, is spreading." The president-elect of the AMA declared in 2003 that "we consider it a crisis when a woman can't find a physician to deliver her baby. We consider it a crisis when a . . . trauma center shuts down, and someone who has been seriously injured in an automobile accident has to be transferred to another hospital. We think there's a meltdown occurring right now."[30]

Concerns about the impact of legal fear on patient care also appeared in popular culture. NBC's hit comedy *Scrubs* offered a stereotypical view of malpractice attorneys as a symbolic enemy in the episode "My Malpractical Decision." Two of the doctors at Sacred Heart Hospital—Perry Cox and John Dorian (J. D.)—found themselves treating the father of Nina Broderick, "the scariest malpractice attorney in the city." The episode reinforced negative stereotypes of trial lawyers, for Ms. Broderick, in the opinion of Dr. Cox, "seemed to create problems where there were none." Physicians and nurses were on edge as she roamed the hallways of Sacred Heart. The cast captured the notion of legal fear among doctors, for, as J. D. noted, "everybody around here had the sense to stay under the radar when Nina Broderick was around."

This episode captured several elements of the narrative of decline used by physicians to frame public debate over the malpractice crisis. Dr. Cox underscored the image of trial lawyers as a symbolic enemy, describing Broderick as "a black haired, soulless bottom feeder." This episode captured the hostility among the medical profession toward malpractice attorneys. Introducing her to J. D., Cox warned, "This woman is pure, molten evil." Cox regarded Broderick with disgust, and asked, "How do you even look at yourself in the mirror, knowing that you are ruining American medicine with frivolous lawsuits?" Although her father was a candidate for an implanted defibrillator to control his cardiac arrhythmia, the doctors let the fear of litigation shape the care of the patient, in effect denying him appropriate care. As Dr. Cox quipped, "Knowing damned well that you'll sue us if anything should go wrong with this *elective* procedure, I'm going to elect *not* to do it." In short, this episode laid the blame for the malpractice crisis squarely at the feet of the legal profession.

During each malpractice crisis, news reports focused particular attention on the plight of pregnant women unable to find accessible prenatal care. Reporters described the struggles of pregnant women who worried that they might have to deliver their babies in unfamiliar surroundings, without the support of their own obstetricians. The struggles of such visible and vulnerable patients personalized the crisis for television audiences. In 1987, for example, *ABC News* described the plight of pregnant women in South Florida who were forced to drive to hospitals up to one hundred miles away in order to deliver their babies. Similar stories reappeared during more recent malpractice crises. In 2002 *Time* profiled a pregnant woman in Arizona forced to pull off the highway to give birth en route to the only maternity ward in a six-thousand-square-mile area. The American College of Obstetricians and Gynecologists warned that 10 percent to 20 percent of all ob-gyns in the United States "either stopped delivering babies, stopped doing gyn surgery or even gave up practice altogether" in response to rising malpractice rates for the profession. This same theme was picked up by President George W. Bush in his 2006 State of the Union address. Bush argued, "Lawsuits are driving many good doctors out of practice—leaving women in nearly 1,500 American counties without a single ob/gyn."[31]

In a related story of decline, news reports warned the public that the threat of malpractice also stifled medical progress. As early as 1971, Michael Halberstam wrote that "instances have been cited in which promising medical or surgical procedures have been abandoned because of their tendency to generate lawsuits." During the California physicians' walkout in 1975, for example, *U.S. News and World Report* warned readers that "many doctors are becoming reluctant to perform hazardous operations, try any procedure that might provide a cure but could be risky. Medical authorities warn that this eventually could stultify progress." The threat of malpractice thus not only burdened physicians, but also jeopardized the availability of new medical treatments for everyone. Such stories of decline were not confined to the popular media, but also appeared in professional publications such as law reviews and medical journals that predicted rising malpractice rates would make it impossible for many doctors to continue practicing medicine.³² Medical dramas underscored the omnipresent fear of lawsuits among clinicians and its impact on clinical decision making. In the sixth season of *Chicago Hope,* for example, one surgeon who went to extraordinary lengths to save the life of a young baseball player was sued when the operation did not succeed. The message of such shows reinforced the notion that despite their best efforts on behalf of patients, doctors who took risks with promising, yet unproven, techniques faced punishment if their efforts failed.

This narrative wove together several complementary threads to build a case for tort reform. In the absence of reform, doctors warned that they would be forced to leave or curtail their practices or relocate to other states. Even for physicians who remained in practice, the constant fear of litigation reshaped medical practice, as doctors avoided "risky" patients who might not fare well with unconventional treatments. Images of patients unable to obtain care from doctors who were trained to treat them, and of women unable to obtain quality prenatal care, painted rising insurance premiums not only as a financial burden, but as a life-threatening condition.

Reformers also contend that the ever-present threat of litigation drives up health care costs. In this story of decline, physicians practice "defensive medicine"—ordering extra, often unnecessary, tests and procedures—to avoid potential litigation. Thus, "legal fear" shapes physicians' treatment decisions and their relationships with patients. Although defensive medicine proved to be hard to define in practice, profiles of doctors who provided "unnecessary" care because of a fear of malpractice suits became commonplace in popular television shows and in political campaigns. Stories of doctors struggling to avoid "frivolous" lawsuits appeared in the first years of the malpractice crisis in the early 1970s. Writing in the *New York Times Magazine* in 1971, Dr. Michael Halberstam described the fear of malpractice as the "doctor's new dilemma." Halberstam wrote, "The very idea of a malpractice suit chills my bones, but it is an idea very hard to get out of my mind, for the frequency of these suits, the size of the judgments rendered, and their effect on medical practice have within the last two years become a constant concern in the medical profession." Halberstam declared that "in my own work I can never quite escape the shadow of malpractice. Although internal medicine has been less plagued by lawsuits than surgery and its sub-specialties, I still live with the subliminal awareness that every phone call, every 'minor' office visit may culminate in a suit." By 1974 the *New York Times* noted that fear of litigation "caused doctors to perform many more laboratory tests and X-rays to back up their diagnoses, should their judgment and treatment be challenged in a court case. These tests increase the cost of medical services."[33]

Similar arguments resurfaced in a variety of forms, and in a variety of settings, over the next four decades. Proponents of tort reform contended that defensive medicine cost "billions of dollars a year to the nation's consumers who in the end must pay for it all." Malpractice premiums accounted for a small proportion of overall health care spending, but physicians argued that the specter of malpractice cast a shadow over every clinical encounter. Even though relatively few patients sued their physicians for malpractice, doctors managed their potential risk by ordering additional tests for *all* patients. As a result, supporters of tort reform claimed that such unnecessary defensive behavior accounted for up to 20 percent of all health care spending.[34]

Political candidates trumpeted the role of malpractice as a cost driver. During the 1992 presidential debate, for example, President George Bush argued that "the medical malpractice people" were responsible for "these frivolous trial-lawyer lawsuits that are running the cost of medical care up by $25 to $50 billion. . . . [I]f you want to help somebody, don't run the costs up by making doctors have to have five or six tests where one would do because of a fear of being sued." The notion that defensive medicine drives up health care spending had strong bipartisan appeal. Bush's opponent in 1992— Arkansas governor Bill Clinton—shared similar concerns about the impact of medical malpractice. Campaigning for his health care reform plan in 1993, Clinton observed that "malpractice not only affects doctors with higher premiums, but a lot of people believe it adds to the cost of the system, because doctors practice what is called defensive medicine and order procedures they otherwise wouldn't just to keep from being sued."[35]

A decade later, similar arguments resurfaced in debates over tort reform. President George W. Bush argued that "the fear of even baseless lawsuits causes good doctors to order excessive tests and procedures and treatments. . . . If you think you're going to get sued, you do everything you possibly can to prevent the trial lawyer from coming after you." As a result, the president warned, "every one of us pays for these awards through higher health care bills." During the contentious debate over health care reform in 2009, Republicans criticized the Obama administration's proposal for failing to address tort reform. Senator John McCain (R-AZ) declared that "any one of our physicians will tell you that they practice defensive medicine, and understandably so, because of their fear of being sued." Senate minority leader Mitch

McConnell (R-KY) echoed these sentiments, arguing that "because of the constant threat of these suits, doctors are forced to order costly but unnecessary tests and procedures just to protect themselves."[36]

Anecdotal examples of defensive medicine appeared frequently in television news coverage of the malpractice crisis. One doctor noted in an interview with *ABC News* in 1985, "I've had to practice defensive medicine, ordering extra tests, extra ultrasounds, extra procedures of any kind. But if you don't do these things and should something go wrong then you have nothing to back you up." Viewers learned that such defensive practices add "$15 to $40 billion a year to the nation's health care bill." As *CBS News* medical consultant Dr. Bob Arnot concluded, "Doctors are going to do defensive medicine to protect themselves from malpractice suits. For instance, you come in and you banged your head. I examine you and find nothing wrong. You feel just fine, but I feel obligated to do a $1,000 brain scan because I don't want to be sued later." More than nine out of ten specialists in Pennsylvania, for example, reported that they ordered additional tests—particularly diagnostic imaging—in "clinically unnecessary circumstances."[37]

Doctors portrayed themselves as the victims of circumstances beyond their control. As caregivers they faced soaring malpractice costs, litigious patients, and "predatory" attorneys. Although physicians' efforts to protect themselves contributed to both higher health care costs and access problems for their patients, these were the unintended consequences of the ever-present fear of litigation. This basic narrative largely defined the nature of public discourse about the medical malpractice crisis for nearly four decades. By defining public discourse about malpractice reform narrowly as an issue of tort reform, however, this narrative avoided the more difficult question of how to improve the quality and reliability of health care services.

A Second Opinion: A Crisis of Quality, Not Liability

Opponents of tort reform argued that physicians and insurers were so preoccupied with the cost of liability coverage that they missed the real malpractice crisis—preventable medical errors. Trial lawyers also challenged the assumptions underlying the policy stories told by physicians and insurers with a new narrative. In this story, "it is not the doctor who needs protection, but the patient."[38] Blame for rising malpractice premiums was placed at the feet of poorly trained or incompetent doctors. For opponents of tort reform, physicians' preferred prescriptions—limiting the right to sue and capping awards for pain and suffering—created unacceptable side effects.

This narrative offered a powerful rebuttal to the cries of crisis in malpractice debates, for it defined the right to sue as a deep-seated American value. In addition, lawyers portrayed malpractice cases as a matter of simple justice, appealing to public beliefs in fair treatment for injured patients and their families. From this vantage point, tort reform did little except limit the ability of injured patients to obtain needed compensation for their economic and medical needs.

Advocates for injured patients described rising malpractice rates as the unavoidable by-product of an epidemic of medical error. "The cause of the malpractice crisis," as the president of the Association of Trial Lawyers of America (ATLA) quipped in 1975, "is malpractice on the part of doctors, and if they want to eliminate the premium problem they should eliminate the malpractice." Trial lawyers rejected calls for tort reform, for in this story, "malpractice is caused by poor medical care, not litigation." Pointing to the pain and suffering of injured patients, opponents of tort reform portrayed malpractice suits as an essential tool to hold "bad doctors" accountable for their actions. The courts, in this narrative, offered justice for those afflicted by medical mistakes. For trial lawyers, the growing number of lawsuits and the rising cost of malpractice coverage were direct consequences of the medical profession's unwillingness, or inability, to discipline its own members. The symbolic power of this diagnosis was based on public fears about medical error. "Patients do not cause malpractice. Lawyers of injured patients do not cause malpractice. It is careless doctors who cause malpractice and thus necessitate premium charges for malpractice insurance." As a Florida attorney interviewed by *ABC News* argued in 1987, "Many doctors are being sued four, five, six, seven times in this community. And they don't have any business practicing medicine."[39]

Stories of dramatic medical mistakes featured prominently in popular television dramas over the past two decades. Television series such as *Boston Legal, Chicago Hope, ER, Grey's Anatomy, The Practice,* and *Scrubs* brought issues of medical malpractice and medical error into millions of homes. The line between news and popular culture became increasingly blurred over time, for reporters often covered health care issues portrayed on television dramas as "real" news. In 1997, for example, the cohost of the *CBS This Morning* news segment observed that she was "watching *Chicago Hope* last night, and last night's episode dealt with a couple of doctors who thought they had something under control and something went terribly wrong."[40] Television medical dramas, which were among the most popular series on network television, reinforced latent concerns about the quality of medical care by highlighting cases of medical malpractice. In addition, by focusing attention on the victims of medical error, such dramas reinforced arguments by attorneys that malpractice reform was a matter not just of insurance rates, but of human lives.

Portraits of physician error occupied a particularly prominent place in NBC's blockbuster drama *ER*. In its fourteen seasons on the air, *ER*'s frenetic pace and graphic images of patient care dramatized how physicians could commit serious, and sometimes deadly, mistakes. In the episode "Do One, Teach One, Kill One," which aired during the second season, an overconfident but still inexperienced Dr. John Carter attempted to biopsy an elderly patient's lung. During the procedure, Carter mistakenly perforated the patient's liver and sent the unfortunate man to the operating room, where he later died in surgery. Carter's first thought after committing the error was not about the patient's welfare, but rather about the impact of his mistake on his own career. Upon realizing his mistake, Carter fumed, "I don't believe this—there goes next year's surgical residency!"

Such portrayals of self-interested, mistake-prone physicians reinforced lawyers' claims that the medical profession was not fully accountable for its mistakes. Furthermore, Carter's fatal error did not produce widespread outrage among the medical staff. His supervising resident, Dr. Peter Benton, reassured Carter that "it happens—it's all right." Carter was counseled that although his experience was painful, "it's how you learn—it'll make you a better doctor." A despondent Carter later complained that both Dr. Benton and the attending surgeon, Dr. Hicks, were so excited to turn his mistake into a chance to perform a difficult and unusual surgery that "they were glad I screwed up." Such story lines underscored the need for patients to press for justice and accountability in the wake of medical mistakes. Television medical dramas also focused public attention on the culture of silence among clinicians by underscoring physicians' reluctance to disclose errors to patients. Trial lawyers argued that many patients sued not for financial gain, but rather to force providers to disclose information about medical mistakes. In the opening episode of the first season of *Scrubs*, the hospital's legal counsel pleaded with the new interns that "if there is a mistake, don't admit it to the patient!"

One of the most vivid portrayals of medical error in a televised medical drama occurred over the first two seasons of *ER*. In the episode "Love's Labor Lost," one of the show's leading characters, Dr. Mark Greene, treated a pregnant woman named Jodi O'Brien. Greene initially suspected that the woman had a bladder infection and discharged her with a prescription for an antibiotic. After suffering a seizure in the hospital parking lot, Mrs. O'Brien returned to the hospital, where she was diagnosed with preeclampsia, a potentially life-threatening condition. With the hospital's obstetrics staff stretched to the limit, Dr. Greene elected to induce labor in the ER and ultimately performed an emergency Caesarean section. Despite the fact that Greene worked all night to save her life, Jodi O'Brien died a traumatic death, calling Greene's judgment into question. This case, which took viewers on a journey from the initial clinical error in judgment through the process of depositions, testimony, and an ultimate settlement with the patient's family, personalized the fear of medical malpractice for millions of viewers.

Stories of fatal medical errors were commonplace in subsequent seasons of *ER*. Malpractice woes continued to dog Dr. Greene, as he faced another wrongful-death suit during the show's fourth season. In season 5, Dr. Elizabeth Corday committed a deadly error after an extended shift; the following year, third-year medical student Abby Lockhart evoked memories of Dr. Carter's early years, as her errors led to a patient's death. Dr. Corday faced another extended malpractice battle during season 7; viewers accompanied her from the initial error through the process of legal depositions and, finally, a settlement. The importance of error as a recurring theme on *ER* reinforced claims by opponents of tort reform that malpractice was a widespread problem and that providers must be held accountable for their mistakes. Doctors' responses to the lawsuits were also instructive, for rather than focusing on the suffering of injured patients and their families, physicians defined malpractice cases as a professional and personal burden. By highlighting the experiences of several of the most prominent characters on the show with medical error and malpractice, producers underscored the widespread presence of error in American medicine. No physician—even a seasoned doctor such as Mark Greene—was immune from making potentially deadly mistakes.[41]

Medical malpractice cases also appeared regularly in popular legal dramas. During the 1990s, dramatic stories of medical error and medical malpractice aired throughout ABC's hit drama *The Practice*. Audiences were introduced to several patients who died after undergoing cosmetic surgeries or other "routine" procedures. In the show's eighth season, viewers followed the case of a grieving husband who blamed his wife's obstetrician for her death during childbirth.[42]

The hit Fox drama *Boston Legal* also introduced audiences to the malpractice debate through the experience of a hypochondriac who sued his primary-care doctor for failing to diagnose or treat his condition. In the episode "An Eye for an Eye," the patient's lawyer, Alan Shore, offered a poignant rebuttal to the notion that his client's claims were "frivolous." The outraged attorney painted a very different picture for the jury:

> Frivolous? Is that what he said? Frivolous? Astonishing. This man who suffers—day in and day out—with migraines so excruciating that he can't work, can't endure ten minutes at his computer, a trained software engineer, and here he is subjecting himself to the laborious and mind-numbing blather of attorneys—for what? Frivolity? For six months, Bill Morgan reached out to his doctor, week after week. Each time, invoiced for thousands and thousands of dollars. And then each time, [he was] dismissed. [His doctor] patted him on the head and sent him on his away. Had Mr. Morgan received the right medical care, or even been directed to a doctor who could have given that care—psychiatric or otherwise—his current state would most likely have been alleviated. But the defendant couldn't be bothered to care.

The message for viewers was clear: patients needed attorneys to intercede for them to obtain needed services or redress for medical mistakes. Ironically, lawyers, not doctors, were portrayed as the champions of patient rights and safety.

News reports also stoked public concerns about medical error by focusing public attention on visible victims of malpractice. Horror stories of serious and fatal medical errors appeared in each debate over malpractice since the 1970s. While most of the media attention during each crisis period focused on the implications of rising malpractice premiums, the stories of decline told by trial lawyers also appeared in news reports. In June 1975, for example, *ABC News* interviewed J. D. Spence, one of the nation's most successful malpractice attorneys. Spence argued that the medical profession had done a poor job of policing itself and that "repeat offenders" represented a continuing threat to patients. Later that month, *NBC News* presented a two-part special report on the malpractice crisis featured differing viewpoints on the controversy over tort reform. In a now familiar argument, lawyers argued the malpractice crisis was the result of an all-too-real threat of malpractice by doctors. The following night, the audience met the family of a young child in Illinois who was awarded $1 million in damages in a malpractice case.[43] Although public attitudes toward the legal profession were not as favorable as they were toward doctors, the right to sue is deeply rooted in American culture and traditions. The notion that "reforms" would prevent injured patients and families from having their day in court allowed opponents to challenge the fundamental fairness of tort reforms, even as the public expressed concerns about the growing litigiousness of American society.

Similar stories of unusual, often fatal, medical errors reappeared in subsequent years, providing a vivid human-interest angle for network news broadcasts. Error was portrayed as a hidden danger lurking behind each health care encounter. As *CBS News* anchor Dan Rather noted in 1995, "Every day in this country people put their lives in the hands of dedicated doctors, nurses, and other professionals who provide the best medical care in the world. But sometimes mistakes are made and things can go terribly wrong. Here in New York, a doctor mistook a patient's dialysis catheter for a feeding tube and ordered food pumped into her abdomen. The patient died. This week, that doctor was sentenced to prison for reckless endangerment." Two years later, *CBS This Morning* described medical errors as a national problem, noting that "in Florida, a patient came out of surgery with the wrong leg amputated. In Pennsylvania, a baby died from receiving the wrong formula. In Arizona, a surgeon sewed a heart valve in upside down."[44] Significantly, media coverage of medical error fixed blame on the behavior of individuals, not institutions.

Heart-wrenching depictions of families coping with the aftermath of medical errors lent a human face to arguments against tort reform. A 2003 report on malpractice presented by *CBS News* illustrated the emotional power of this narrative. Reporters described the case of a toddler who died after a visit to the emergency room. "Three days after his second birthday, Owen Gardner died at the hands of medical professionals his parents trusted. . . . The Gardners are part of an emotional debate on Capitol Hill: whether pain and suffering damages in medical malpractice cases should be limited. The Gardners, backed by trial lawyers, say you just can't put a price on human life." In 2003 *Good Morning America* sought to "put a face to the debate" over President Bush's proposal to cap medical malpractice awards at $250,000. Diane Sawyer introduced viewers to Heather Lewinsky, "a little girl scarred for life when a doctor performed radical and improper surgery on her." During her interview, the "scarred, scared teen" urged lawmakers to reject a proposed cap on pain and suffering awards. As she told the audience, "I totally missed my childhood because of what the doctor did. I think I should be able to have an adulthood."[45] Such vivid tales of patients who had suffered grievous injuries offered a powerful rebuttal to supporters of tort reform who railed against "frivolous" lawsuits.

Trial lawyers also challenged the notion that rising liability insurance premiums represented a crisis for physicians. The president of the Trial Lawyers of America dismissed the California physicians' strike in 1975 as a publicity stunt that was a part of a "multi-million dollar propaganda campaign." A decade later, the president of the New York State Trial Lawyers Association echoed this theme, describing the malpractice "crisis" as "a phony issue created by doctors." This alternative diagnosis placed blame for rising malpractice premiums squarely at the feet of the medical profession; since error was widespread in medicine, the high cost of liability insurance was the direct result of doctors' own actions. As the president of the New York State Trial Lawyers Association argued in 1975, "People in high positions in the medical profession are trying to create a crisis so they can abolish malpractice suits. Then they can kill anybody and it won't make any difference." As one representative from the Association of Trial Lawyers of America argued in 1975, "Litigation has a therapeutic effect. Liability breeds care." Furthermore, lawyers rejected the notion that rising malpractice rates had created a crisis of access for patients. As one Florida attorney noted, "The emergency room situation is a hoax. Every doctor is saying that if I treat somebody I'm going to get sued. Well, that isn't true—he has to do something wrong."[46] Efforts to limit doctors' liability for medical errors, from this vantage point, merely fostered substandard care and decreased providers' accountability for their actions.

In addition, opponents of tort reform described it as a painful prescription with serious side effects. Lawyers argued that tort reforms such as caps on damages for pain and suffering merely punished the victims of medical error by undermining the ability of patients to receive proper compensation for their injuries. In 1985, for example, the Association of Trial Lawyers of America complained that doctors' pleas for malpractice reforms would create "a special niche in American law be carved out for doctors, while the rest of us are held responsible for our carelessness under time-tested rules of law." Lawyers employed their own story of decline, describing doctors' support for tort reform as a thinly veiled attempt to strip patients of their constitutional rights and avoid responsibility for the consequences of their mistakes. By 1986 the executive director of the ATLA argued, "We're dealing with vast numbers of people who are having significant rights taken away from them by state legislators." This same theme reappeared in each subsequent debate over tort reform. After the Obama administration authorized the use of state-level experiments on liability reform and patient safety, the American Association of Justice declared that "it is critical that these demonstration projects preserve Americans' Seventh Amendment right to a trial by jury.... [A]ny efforts to limit patients' rights are not acceptable."[47]

Opponents of tort reform described limits on the size of jury awards in malpractice cases as a dangerous precedent. During the debate over Amendment 10, a tort-reform proposal introduced as a ballot initiative in Florida in 1988, lawyers urged citizens to "not vote to deprive themselves of their right to recover just compensation for their loss of the ability to fully enjoy life from those persons or corporations that negligently bring about their injuries." For opponents of damage caps, the campaign to control malpractice costs threatened the independence and discretion of juries. "The battle over [Amendment 10] is not for the purpose of eliminating unjustified lawsuits or excessive verdicts. It is an attempt, to a large extent, to eliminate the jury system in this state." Similar arguments reappeared in malpractice debates around the nation in recent decades. As the president of the West Virginia Trial Lawyers Association argued in 2002, "The real threat that we face is to our system of justice. They [reformers] want to take away our fundamental right to seek and obtain compensation for a wrong."[48]

In a similar fashion, opponents of tort reform also challenged the notion that defensive medicine contributed to rampant health care inflation. As one of the nation's leading malpractice lawyers noted in an interview with *People* in 1978, "All that such tests mean is that a doctor lacks confidence in his own abilities. I never had one case based on a doctor not ordering an X-ray or a test. If they spent half as much time studying medical books as they do figuring out ways to hide their income, they wouldn't have to worry about malpractice." Lawyers argued that "medicine ought to be defensive, as should every profession." The solution to rising medical malpractice costs, therefore, "is for doctors to practice better medicine, not to reduce the rights of their victims."[49]

Malpractice attorneys also claimed that they were unfairly scapegoated for rising malpractice costs. In recent decades, the term *trial lawyer* became an epithet in policy discourse. Trial lawyers became a symbolic enemy in the crisis narratives told by physicians. Doctors argued that attorneys had a powerful financial incentive to file unwarranted or inappropriate lawsuits. Attorneys in malpractice cases are typically paid on a contingency basis, where their fees are based upon a percentage of the final settlement or jury award. Trial attorneys rejected the claim that contingency fees encouraged a proliferation of "frivolous" lawsuits. Instead, opponents of tort reform defended the practice in the 1970s, arguing that it provided "a key for the poor man to the courthouse doors." The contingency system allowed patients to obtain legal representation without an up-front payment. As the president of the New York State Trial Lawyers Association argued in 1984, "Without trial lawyers, the maimed and disabled would not be compensated by those responsible." Two decades later, the legal community repeated this defense of contingency fees. In 2005 one of the nation's leading malpractice attorneys complained that "[President] Bush makes it sound like every lawsuit that is brought is junk or frivolous. But we do everything we can to weed out cases that are without merit. We have to. Our own money is at risk."[50]

The policy narratives offered by opponents of tort reform, however, remain incomplete. Attorneys offered no plausible prescription of their own to address rising malpractice insurance rates. In particular, trial lawyers failed to acknowledge the impact of legal fear on quality-improvement initiatives. As Senators Hillary Rodham Clinton (D-NY) and Barack Obama (D-IL) wrote in the *New England Journal of Medicine*, "The current tort system does not promote open communication to improve patient safety." The threat of litigation has a corrosive effect on efforts to improve the quality of health care, for in the current culture of blame, fear of being sued discourages doctors from disclosing adverse events. To date, the principal roadblocks to meaningful malpractice reform are rhetorical, for although the policy narratives told by doctors and lawyers are partially true, each suffers from critical sins of omission. The resulting lack of consensus hinders efforts to enact practical reforms that will improve patient safety and save lives. As Senators Hillary Clinton and Barack Obama argued in 2006, "Instead of focusing on the few areas of intense disagreement, such as the possibility of mandating caps on the financial damages awarded to patients," reformers must "focus on a more fundamental issue: the need to improve patient safety."[51]

A New Road Map for Reform

The seeds of a new policy narrative have lain dormant beneath the surface of public debates since the early 1970s. As Michael Halberstam noted in 1971, "At almost every step in medical practice, better communications among regulating groups, more effective sanctions, and continual re-certifications of competence are required. Only after these steps are taken will medicine have occasion to be righteously indignant about the frequency of malpractice suits."[52] Instead of fearmongering, reformers must tell a new story that unites rather than divides doctors, lawyers, and patients around shared interests and values. Such a story would engage the public with familiar themes of tragedy (preventable deaths), heroes (dedicated clinicians and researchers), and technological progress (electronic medical records, computerized physician order entry, bar coding). This new narrative weaves well-established public beliefs in medical progress and the power of technology into a story of progress and shared security.

Elements of such a new policy narrative focused on patient safety are already in place, as discussions of medical errors have become commonplace in news coverage, on television medical dramas, and in popular culture in recent years. The magnitude of preventable medical error is well documented. Each year, more Americans die from medical errors than from motor vehicle crashes, breast cancer, and AIDS. The publication of the Institute of Medicine's landmark report *To Err Is Human,* in particular, attracted widespread media attention over the past decade, raising public awareness of the widespread scope of medical error in the American health care system. The report's estimate that medical errors caused between forty-four and ninety-eight thousand deaths each year was widely reported by print and broadcast media and also sparked a flurry of activity among doctors, hospitals, and other providers to explore new avenues to improve patient safety. Even using the more conservative lower estimate, medical error represents the eighth leading cause of death in the nation. As the *Journal of the American Medical Association* editorialized in 1998, "Modern health care represents the most complex safety challenge of any activity on earth. However, we have failed to design our systems for safety, relying instead on requiring individual error-free performance enforced by punishment." Unlike other high-risk industries—such as aviation and automobiles—health care providers have been slow to embrace systemic approaches to quality improvement.[53] In large part, this is a consequence of the rhetoric of crisis, for by focusing public attention on greedy lawyers and bad doctors, reformers targeted the behavior of individuals, not the design of organizations, as the principal contributors to malpractice.

In many respects, television doctors have been more forthcoming about error, and more accepting of the need for disclosure, than their real-life counterparts. During the fourth season of the hit comedy *Scrubs,* Dr. Perry Cox, an attending physician at the fictional Sacred Heart Hospital, observed that error is inevitable in medical practice. In the episode "My First Kill," Cox deadpanned that "each and every one of you is going to kill a patient. At some point in your residency you will screw up, they will die, and it will be burned into your conscience forever." After this lecture, J. D., the series' leading character, shied away from ordering any risky procedures for patients, lest he inadvertently kill his first patient. This avoidance strategy, however, soon prompted a new conversation with Dr. Cox, who told J. D. that "fear is good—it keeps you from becoming a crappy doctor."

As Victoria Rideout demonstrated in her analysis of *Grey's Anatomy* as a health educator, information presented in television shows shapes the behavior of audiences long after a show airs; as many as one in six viewers sought more information about a health topic, or visited a doctor or other health provider, about something they first saw on *Grey's Anatomy*. The sixth season of *Grey's Anatomy* highlighted the potential of medical dramas to educate the public about the causes of medical error. In the episode "I Saw What I Saw," the death of a patient led the chief of medicine, Dr. Richard Webber, to conduct an investigation to affix blame and responsibility for the incident. Several residents and attending physicians cared for the patient, who suffered from what appeared to be minor burns, in the wake of a mass casualty at an area hotel. After assembling bits and pieces of the evening's events, the hospital's senior physicians realized that the patient's death was due to a series of seemingly innocuous missteps and missed handoffs. Her death was preventable, for it resulted from poor communication—in the chaotic environment of the ER, no physician claimed responsibility for her care; although six different doctors treated her, each was distracted, and no one took the time to properly assess the patient. As Dr. Derek Sheppard observed, the death revealed flaws in the hospital's own processes and training systems: "Maybe it wasn't one doctor. Maybe it was too many doctors, too many doctors that don't trust each other." The fact that no doctor willingly took responsibility for this patient is what Atul Gawande terms "silent disengagement," as each physician focused only on their own specialized domain. This episode underscored the principal findings of the report *To Err Is Human*, which noted that "the majority of medical errors do not result from individual recklessness or the actions of a particular group. . . . More commonly, errors are caused by faulty systems, processes, and conditions that lead people to make mistakes or fail to prevent them."[54]

Celebrities also became narrators of the need to improve patient safety in recent years, underscoring the tragedy of preventable medical errors in film and in the media. After a medication error nearly took the lives of his new-born twins in 2007, Dennis Quaid became a tireless patient-safety advocate. Speaking before the National Press Club, he declared, "My mission today is to drive awareness . . . awareness of both the harm and the opportunity to save countless lives."[55] Drawing upon his experience in Hollywood, Quaid produced a documentary, *Chasing Zero: Winning the War on Healthcare Harm,* which premiered at the 2010 Global Patient Safety Summit. The film reached a national audience later that year on the Discovery Channel. His efforts represent a promising new approach to addressing the malpractice morass, for documentaries emerged as a powerful tool to raise public aware-ness of important policy issues from global warming (*An Inconvenient Truth*) to health care reform (*Sicko*) and public education (*Waiting for Superman*) over the past decade. As a tragic story of senseless deaths, Quaid's work dem-onstrates how reformers might employ "human interest" stories with visible victims to engage average citizens in debates over malpractice reform.

Meaningful malpractice reform requires the creation of policies that will encourage the development of "high-reliability organizations" in health care. As James Reason notes, debates about malpractice reform stress individual responsibility; both malpractice suits and hospitals' internal mortality and morbidity conferences focus on providers who deviate from established norms of practice (that is, "bad apples"). Medical mistakes—whether or not they result in injury—are "sentinel events" that expose underlying quality problems that result in death or injury to patients. Errors are often latent in health care systems as a result of financial constraints, insufficient staffing, inadequate training, or time pressures. In this context, successful reform, as Lawrence Gostin argues, "requires designing processes and systems to pre-vent human error, rather than focusing on blame." Recent research on medi-cal error, therefore, undermines the credibility of the "bad apples" view of medical malpractice offered by trial lawyers, for physicians rarely commit errors in isolation.[56]

This new narrative builds upon long-standing public beliefs in medical progress and the power of technology to improve daily life. Technological advances—as embodied in electronic medical records, "smart" pumps for delivering medicines, and computerized order entry for pharmaceuticals—can significantly reduce preventable errors. As the American Hospital Asso-ciation noted in a national advertising campaign in 2009, "Doctors, nurses, and other health care professionals have been changing the way they deliver care in an effort to make care better and safer. . . . [H]ospitals are harnessing the power of information technology and using bar codes to ensure the right medicine goes to the right patient at the right time."[57] In short, a growing body of work on medical error and quality improvement supports the narrative fidelity of this story of progress.

Anesthesiology, in particular, offers a powerful lesson about the prospects of improving patient safety for contemporary reformers. In the mid-1980s, anesthesiologists faced spiraling medical malpractice rates; the field was one of the riskiest areas of medical practice in terms of professional liability. News coverage highlighted horror stories of healthy patients undergoing routine surgery. In response, anesthesiologists engaged in a critical self-assessment of professional practices, drawing upon patient data that indicated when errors were most likely to occur during surgery. Working with medical device manufacturers, nurses, and other stakeholders, physicians identified the leading causes of error and developed a professional consensus about how to improve the process of care. In addition to saving lives, these efforts also reduced the frequency and cost of malpractice claims. By the mid-1990s, the rate of preventable errors plummeted, and claims for anesthesia-related deaths and disability declined. Anesthesia became the only medical specialty to achieve a "six-sigma" level of quality, with fewer than four deaths per million patients. As a result, the average premiums for liability insurance paid by anesthesiologists in 2002 were comparable to those in the mid-1980s.[58]

A key advantage of this story of progress over the existing rhetoric of crisis is that reforms can be developed by doctors' and hospitals' professional groups and implemented by providers themselves. The unique accrediting role of the Joint Commission on the Accreditation of Healthcare Organizations provides leverage for reform-minded providers, as documented lifesaving practices can ultimately be incorporated into accreditation standards. Policy makers can champion the cause of patient safety through a new story of progress, while reserving detailed discussions for key stakeholders. Such efforts to improve patient safety are already taking root, including the adoption of surgical checklists similar to those used by airline pilots and the use of mandatory "time-outs" to lower the risk of wrong-site surgeries.[59]

In the seventh season of Grey's Anatomy, efforts to prevent medical errors took center stage in the episode "I Will Survive." Dr. April Kepner—who played a critical role in the previous season's preventable-death case—won the enmity of her fellow residents by promoting the use of a checklist to improve patient care. Dr. Kepner succinctly summarized the rationale for the new initiative, noting that "it's based on a protocol used in aviation; a simple checklist has led to a huge drop in plane crashes." After one of the attending physicians, Dr. Hunt, endorsed the idea, Kepner faced indifference and hostility as she sought to persuade her fellow physicians to incorporate the idea into their daily practice. This episode underscored both the possibilities and the pitfalls inherent in efforts to improve patient safety, capturing the same struggles described by Atul Gawande in *The Checklist Manifesto*.[60]

Providers also pioneered new approaches to averting malpractice suits in recent years by embracing the power of apology; the University of Michigan's "Sorry Works" program, for example, significantly reduced the frequency and cost of malpractice suits by requiring physicians and hospital administrators to fully disclose, and apologize for, any medical errors that occurred during a patient stay. In 2009 Sandra Coletta, the president and CEO of Kent Hospital in Warwick, Rhode Island, attracted national attention after she apologized to actor James Woods and his family for his brother's death in the hospital emergency room. Colletta's candor illustrates the power of providers to lead the campaign for quality improvement and underscores the importance of honest, open communication to improved patient safety. Speaking to the media, she declared, "We know we're not perfect at Kent Hospital. Mistakes were made. We can do better." In the wake of her action, the Woods family not only dropped its lawsuit against the hospital, but also funded a new institute to improve patient safety.[61] These cases illustrate not only that compromise is possible in heated debates over malpractice, but that collaboration offers a way forward for both providers and patients.

Overcoming the rhetorical roadblocks that stymied past debates about medical malpractice reform may require a change of venue. Since the mid-1970s, debates over malpractice reform occurred primarily within state legislatures. Debates about malpractice reform fostered the mobilization of resources by private interests, who defined the conversation through media blitzes, letter-writing campaigns, and rallies. Legislators focused their attention on limiting punitive damages and other incremental tort reforms.[62] The legislative setting is ill-equipped to foster political deliberation where parties puzzle through clinical data, patient stories, and policy options. Furthermore, the public spotlight of legislative debates discourages parties from risk taking. To move the debate forward, legislators may need to step aside.

Secure, private negotiations among key stakeholders offer a better prospect of nurturing a deliberative approach to liability reform. In such an environment, stakeholders could speak freely and explore areas of mutual concern, without fear that such conversations will be portrayed as a betrayal of group interests. Voluntary participation in such conversations will encourage stakeholders to "think out loud" and discover common ground in a nurturing environment, in contrast to the charged environment of many "blue-ribbon" commissions, where testimony in public hearings is an exercise in posturing, not problem solving. The principal goal of this new approach is to lay the foundation for an ongoing, evolutionary conversation among stakeholders.

Policy makers must change their strategy to bring physicians, patients, and other health professionals to join together to fight a common enemy. Supporters of reform should embrace a classic narrative of progress that celebrates innovation and risk taking. Stories of the courage and perseverance of providers who commit themselves to eradicating error, despite the financial cost and risk of doing so, add a heroic element to malpractice debates. These stories also harness the emotional appeal of visible victims and have a strong sense of narrative coherence, for they build on the real-life experiences of hospitals, surgeons, and other providers.

This new policy narrative appeals to both the common good and economic self-interest. Medical error, in short, has no defenders. In the 1950s, for example, political leaders used the successful launch of Sputnik—the first satellite to orbit Earth—as a call to action to mobilize support for the "space race." In the wake of Sputnik, for example, efforts to upgrade the nation's scientific research establishment were redefined as a matter of national security, leading to the passage of educational reforms and increased spending on research. By developing a new narrative of progress, reformers can reshape the rhetoric of reform, building common ground among a group of strange bedfellows that includes physicians, insurers, patients, and the legal profession. Writing in 2010, Dennis Quaid argued, "The true battle being waged in patient safety is between fear and hope."[63] It will take sustained leadership to repair the damage done by decades of crisis talk, but a new narrative to address the chronic problems plaguing the malpractice system has the potential to mobilize support for well-established yet currently underutilized error-reduction techniques that will both save lives and limit the financial burden of medical malpractice insurance for providers.

CHAPTER FOUR

The Nurse Staffing Crisis

The impending crisis in nurse staffing has the potential to impact the very health and security of our society.
—Joint Commission on Accreditation of Healthcare Organizations, *Health Care at the Crossroads: Strategies for Addressing the Evolving Nursing Crisis*

There has been a shortage of nurses for years, but now the situation has reached critical condition.
—Wyatt Andrews, "Nursing Shortage May Be Putting Lives at Risk," *CBS Evening News,* May 24, 2006

CONTEMPORARY DISCUSSIONS of the nursing shortage bear an uncanny resemblance to earlier warnings of a nurse staffing crisis over the past half century. American hospitals faced similar nurse staffing shortfalls on several occasions since the 1940s. Hospital administrators, nurses, and public officials framed each nursing shortage using cries of crisis. Although some observers argue that the contemporary nursing shortage is fundamentally different from those in the past, the way Americans talk about the supply of nurses has changed little over the past five decades.[1]

As a political symbol, the nursing crisis plays on public anxieties. Illness is a stressful time for most individuals and their families. Crisis talk targeted the fears of vulnerable patients and families who worried that care would not be available when they were sick or unable to care for themselves. Each time the nursing labor market tightened, reformers employed stories of decline to build support for recruiting nurses by citing worrisome trends, making dire predictions, and highlighting the plight of visible victims whose care was compromised by the nursing shortage. The common element in these stories—and, indeed, the connective tissue in narratives of crisis—was fear. Crisis narratives portrayed each emerging shortage as a matter of life or death, warning that sick patients might not receive lifesaving care in their most desperate hour.

Each time the nursing shortage in American hospitals became acute, talk of an emerging crisis reinforced the notion that the health care system had reached a "tipping point." Reformers painted a bleak picture of the future unless dramatic steps were taken. In recent years, advocates for reform described the nursing shortage as "a 'perfect storm' brewing. We have aging nurses and aging nursing faculties. We have fewer people choosing to come into nursing . . . and we have millions of baby-boomers whose health needs will grow exponentially."[2] In this story, nurses were innocent victims of circumstances beyond their control. Heart-wrenching profiles of nurses in newspapers, nightly news programs, and periodic "special reports" on television all reported different variations of the same crisis story: too few nurses caring for too many patients.

More than 750 nursing strikes have been recorded in recent decades, making nursing among the most strike-prone professions in the United States. In the spring of 2010, more than twelve thousand nurses in Minneapolis–St. Paul staged a one-day strike—the largest nursing walkout in US history—to protest staffing levels in Minnesota hospitals. Carrying signs demanding "Safe Staffing Now" nurses described understaffed hospitals as a threat to the quality of care for all patients. Although hospital administrators dismissed such claims and argued that nurses' demands were both unaffordable and unnecessary, striking nurses maintained that their actions were designed to protect the public from unsafe care. As one union leader declared, "They've had enough. It's time to say that we're going to do what we have to do to protect our patients." After a tense standoff that lasted for weeks, the Minnesota Nurses Association agreed to a new contract that provided modest wage increases and preserved existing health and retirement benefits, but abandoned its call for mandatory nurse-staffing ratios.[3]

Public deliberation about nurse staffing illustrates Wittgenstein's notion that "we are misled by the imagery embedded in our language." Repeated warnings of a nursing crisis failed to resonate with the public, for during each shortage the overwhelming majority of Americans continued to receive high-quality care, and few patients were denied treatment or turned away because of a lack of nurses. To address the ongoing and recurring shortage of nurses in an aging society, reformers must first cut through the conceptual clutter used in public debates about nurse staffing. To do so, reformers must follow Wittgenstein's prescription to begin not by "giving new information, but by arranging what we have always known."[4] The recurring shortage of nurses is cyclical in nature, but it is exacerbated by cries of crisis that define the shortage as a short-term, acute problem.

The consequences of this confusion are not trivial, for in describing the nursing shortage as an acute crisis, reformers missed an opportunity to tell a different and more powerful policy story. An underlying—yet undeveloped—narrative during each crisis period offered a more fruitful path to building long-term public support for investments in nursing education and improved working conditions. Policy makers and nurses sought to raise awareness of the contributions of nurses to patient safety. This narrative viewed additional spending on nurses—either by expanding training programs or by improving nursing pay—as a worthwhile investment in better health care.

Constructing the Nursing Crisis

The notion of an emerging crisis in nurse staffing can be traced back to the mid-1940s. The end of World War II brought a surge in hospital utilization; admissions to hospitals increased by more than one million patients from 1945 to 1946. As 1945 drew to a close, doctors in New York warned that the nursing shortage "has for all practical purposes reached the stage of an emergency." Although early estimates of the nursing shortage were imprecise, news reports noted that "anyone who visits a hospital anywhere can see there aren't enough nurses." Even though more nurses were employed than ever before, news reports described a widespread and worsening staffing crisis in American hospitals. By 1947 nine states had convened conferences to address the "critical nursing shortage," and the American Hospital Association reported that more than thirty-three thousand hospital beds were unavailable to patients because of a lack of nursing personnel.[5]

In the 1940s and 1950s, the nursing shortage was linked to the rapid expansion of the nation's hospital industry. The Hospital Survey and Construction Act of 1946, also known as the Hill-Burton Act, provided federal grants in aid to states to subsidize the expansion and renovation of hospitals around the nation. The Hill-Burton program contributed to a steady growth in hospital capacity, as the number of hospitals increased from 6,125 in 1946 to 7,156 in 1975. At the same time, the expansion of private health insurance coverage lowered barriers to the use of hospital services. As more insured patients sought care at a growing number of hospitals around the nation, the demand for nurses rose substantially. The number of nurses practicing in New York State, for example, increased by fifty-five thousand in the decade following the end of World War II, yet one-third of the state's nursing positions remained vacant in 1954.[6]

Nursing shortages were a recurring problem in the 1960s and 1970s. By 1974 four thousand nurses in northern California went on strike, demanding higher wages, improved working conditions, and more participation in hospital governance. The strike closed dozens of hospitals in the region. Strikers paralyzed local hospitals, as the California Nurses Association declared that "we will no longer staff hospital areas while supervisory and other non-striking personnel are free to undertake non-acute or non-emergency care." The three-week walkout attracted national media attention, as many hospitals found it impossible to properly staff emergency departments and intensive care units. As a result, hospital officials in the region declared that the strike "brings a genuine health care crisis to San Francisco. Most of the patients aren't in intensive care units unless they're fighting for their lives." Although doctors, hospital administrators, and some nurses criticized the picketers for "irresponsible" behavior that placed patients at risk, both the American Nurses Association and the Teamsters' Union supported the nurses' actions. After intervention by a federal mediator, nurses won retroactive salary increases of nearly 11 percent, pledges from hospitals to include nurses in patient-care planning and unit-staffing discussions, and more flexible scheduling.[7]

Media coverage in the early 1980s repeated familiar warnings of a worsening crisis. Desperate hospitals offered nurses higher salaries and signing bonuses in a frantic attempt to keep their doors open. Television news reports profiled hospitals struggling to hire enough nurses and overworked nurses at risk of burnout. News broadcasts informed viewers in 1981 that "there's now a growing shortage of qualified nurses in this country and that shortage is about to become a crisis in health care." As hospitals struggled to care for a growing number of sicker patients with fewer nurses, the remaining nurses were stretched thin. Nurses, as *ABC News* warned, "are leaving the profession. There are 1,400,000 registered nurses in the United States, but only 600,000 are working full time and U.S. hospitals report 100,000 nursing vacancies."[8]

Each nursing shortage was framed as an acute threat to the public. Although the number of nurses had reached an all-time high in the late 1980s, "hospitals and nursing homes still need at least 150,000 more nurses." By 1987 the *New York Times* informed readers that the nursing profession "faced the most severe shortage in its history" and that "the critical shortage of registered nurses . . . is expected to grow even larger in the future." Images of a "sudden" and "dangerous" shortage spreading like an epidemic across the nation fueled public concern. As one senior executive at the American Hospital Association noted, "Never before have there been nurse shortages in every single state, in every kind of clinical area."[9] Narratives of crisis described each successive nursing shortage as more widespread and severe than those in the past.

The symbolic power of crisis narratives drew upon the proximity of nursing as a profession for patients and families. As the primary caregivers for millions of patients in hospitals, nursing homes, and home health care settings, nurses were highly respected and familiar figures for most Americans. In any given year, "nearly every person's health care experience involves the contribution of a registered nurse."[10] Because nursing strikes often led hospitals to cancel surgeries and curtail elective admissions and diagnostic tests, otherwise healthy patients also worried that their own access to health care services would be disrupted by the emerging crisis. Furthermore, since most Americans will visit a doctor's office, clinic, or hospital for care at some point each year, all patients may consider themselves to be "at risk" from the effects of the shortage.

By the end of the 1980s, hospitals resorted to desperate measures to recruit and retain nursing staff. Some institutions offered "bounties" of one thousand dollars or more to bring in new nurses, while others lured recruits with bonuses of leased cars or ski lessons. Amid talk of a critical shortage, employment agencies charged hospitals up to ten thousand dollars for successful nursing placements. Growing competition among hospitals to hire nurses created "haves" and "have-nots," as hospitals that could afford to pay higher salaries filled their positions by luring nurses from other institutions. The end result, as the *Times* editorialized, was a "crippling shortage of nurses" in American hospitals at the end of the 1980s.[11]

Similar cries of a worsening nursing crisis reappeared after 2000. With more than 126,000 vacant nursing positions across the nation in 2001, media coverage warned the public about the urgent need for more nurses. News reports focused particular attention on how the shortage would impact care for vulnerable patients. *NBC News* described an "alarming shortage of registered nurses, especially those with critical care training. The problems are only getting worse." State legislators in New York described the state's nursing shortage as a "death spiral," and labor leaders argued that "this is a crisis for all New Yorkers, of every age group in every capacity." Talk of crisis persisted in recent years. By 2006 *CBS News* warned viewers of "the growing threat posed by a shortage of nursing staff." A year later *NBC News* also described the "serious shortage" as a "threat to public health." Reporters described the scope of the problem in ominous terms, noting that "the nursing shortage is one of the most dangerous aspects of American health care."[12]

Over the past decade, televised medical dramas such as *Grey's Anatomy* also highlighted the nursing shortage for millions of viewers. In 2006 the show dedicated several episodes to explore the concerns of nurses at Seattle Grace Hospital. In a significant departure from the physician-centered plot-line of the show's first season, the episode "Break on Through" featured angry, frustrated nurses who stood outside the hospital chanting, "Fair hours, fair wages! Fair hours, fair wages!" Doctors fended for themselves as the nursing staff walked a picket line outside. Concerns about working conditions lay at the heart of the dispute between the hospital and its nursing staff. Irate nurses confronted Dr. Richard Webber, the hospital's chief of medicine, declaring that "we are overworked and exhausted!" Outside, protesters decried both mandatory overtime and extended shifts by holding picket signs that read, "Overtime Kills!" and "Nurses Are Overworked and Understaffed!" The chief expressed sympathy for the nurses' demands, but for the hospital the strike was ultimately a matter of dollars and cents. "We need an additional forty nurses to relieve the overtime they are striking about," Webber declared. "That's two million dollars a year we don't have."

Nurses defined the emerging crisis using two distinct stories of decline to frame public discourse about the crisis of nurse staffing. First, nurses argued that the shortage of caregivers would limit access to needed care. Second, nurses painted a doomsday scenario for the future, warning that future generations would face a pervasive, and urgent, shortage of trained nurses. In each crisis narrative, the short-term and long-term prospects for the nursing profession are bleak.

Diminished Access to Care

During each nursing shortage from the 1940s to the present day, nurses and the media warned that hospitals would be forced to limit services or turn away patients in need of care. In the 1940s, for example, the National Nursing Council reported that without enough nurses, many hospitals had no choice but to close wards or curtail admissions. Similar warnings reappeared in the early 1960s. "The shortage of professionally trained R.N.s," physicians complained, "is limiting the usefulness of hospital facilities throughout our land and adding immeasurably to the cost of health care. It is common for patients to have to wait for hospital beds when parts of the hospital are closed for lack of nurses." The critical shortage of nurses represented a significant access barrier for patients. As the *New York Times* noted, the "shortage in private hospitals means that available nurses are overburdened, that hospital beds must remain unoccupied, and that operating theatres must be run on short schedules."[13] The message for the public was clear: the nursing shortage represented a clear and present danger for anyone needing hospital services.

Media coverage of the nursing crisis during the late 1970s and early 1980s presented viewers with horror stories of tragic patient complications or even deaths resulting from insufficient staffing. In one high-profile case, a stabbing victim at Lincoln Hospital in the South Bronx died because no operating room was available; without enough nurses, the hospital was forced to trim services. The scope of the crisis, furthermore, affected all Americans and was not confined to one state or region. New reports noted that "every United States hospital needs nurses," but "hospital beds are being cut back, operating rooms are being closed, and critical care services reduced because there are not enough nurses. This nationwide nursing shortage is particularly severe and dangerous in intensive care units, a growing part of modern health care."[14] Crisis narratives warned that the acute shortage placed lives at risk, for despite the proliferation of promising new treatments and therapies, patients still needed nurses at the bedside. Indeed, the advent of new medical technologies placed more, not fewer, demands on nurses.

During each nursing shortage, news reports focused particular attention on the sickest and most vulnerable patients. Horror stories described patients waiting for hours in emergency department corridors because no nurses were available to staff medical-surgical floors and overworked nurses responsible for managing scores of patients on late-night shifts. The nursing shortage forced hospitals to care for the sick and injured under "battlefield conditions." As one PBS special report noted in 1988, "When beds fill up in critical care, patients are turned away." The president of the American Nurses Association echoed this same theme, arguing that "there are hospitals that are unable to schedule surgeries on a timely basis. There are emergency rooms that are going on diversion because they are very busy and there may not be adequate numbers of registered nurses . . . where many patients may need to be admitted."[15]

Similar stories of substandard care featured prominently in more recent debates over nurse staffing. At hearings before the US Senate in 2001, the president of the American Organization of Nurse Executives testified, "We have beds, and in some cases entire care units in intensive care closed, neonatal units closed, medical and surgical beds closed." As a result, she noted, "surgical schedules have been canceled. We have major backups in all of our emergency rooms. Sometimes we have patients staying 36 hours in emergency rooms because of the inability to get them a patient care bed." Crisis narratives focused particular attention on the state of emergency care. By 2003 the nursing shortage remained dire. Viewers of *60 Minutes* learned that the "severe and dangerous shortage of nurses" meant that "emergency rooms are shutting down, surgeries are delayed, and most disturbing of all, patients are sometimes not getting the critical care they desperately need." After an unattended patient died in a Los Angeles hospital emergency room in 2007, news stories decried the state of emergency care and the loss of compassion in American hospitals. Reporters described the case as "just representative of what's happening in the emergency medical system as a whole. . . . [T]he system is overtaxed and it's at its brink. And it's because there are nursing shortages." *NBC News* briefed viewers in 2007 on "an emergency inside America's emergency rooms. A new survey shows doctors believe patients are dying because of overcrowded, overburdened ERs." NBC's medical correspondent turned to a familiar metaphor, comparing the situation facing patients needing urgent care to "almost a perfect storm: not enough emergency rooms, fewer hospital beds, a nursing shortage."[16]

An Uncertain Future

A related story of decline describes the present nursing shortage as a harbinger of things to come. The crippling shortage of nurses, in such narratives, not only threatens care for current patients, but also casts a shadow over future generations. Analyzing current trends in the nursing labor force—from the age of the nursing workforce to impending retirements of older nurses—reformers warned that current trends placed the profession itself at risk. News reports offered a dire forecast of a future without caregivers. Dire predictions of the future of nursing as a profession are not new. In the early 1950s, the *New York Times* cautioned readers, "There is every indication that the shortage will become 'more critical,' 'more severe,' and 'more acute' in the near future."[17] Each time concerns about an acute nursing shortage appeared on the policy agenda, reformers called for immediate action to expand nursing education to fill the gap. Episodic shortfalls in nurse staffing, however, recurred on several occasions from the 1950s to the present.

By 2000 news stories described a worsening shortage with no end in sight. Reporters warned audiences that "the nursing shortage is spreading nationwide. Ninety-four percent of hospitals in the west have declared or expect a shortage, 82 percent in the Northeast, 75 percent in the Midwest." Estimates of future shortages were sobering, if not alarming. "The biggest concern is for the future. Projections are that in 20 years, the country will have 20 percent fewer nurses than it needs." For reformers, the shortage of nurses was a matter of life and death, as hospital administrators noted that the challenge of staffing hospitals would grow more acute each year. "The nation is currently engulfed in a huge nursing shortage, which is going to get worse. The baby boomers are long since inured to the idea that when they retire, nobody is going to want to give them Social Security. But they may not have been informed that when they get old and go into a hospital, there will probably not be anyone on the ward who's authorized to dole out medication."[18]

During each nursing shortage, news reports and studies offered unsettling predictions of a continuing crisis. In 2002 two leading national health policy organizations—the Robert Wood Johnson Foundation and the Joint Commission on Accreditation of Healthcare Organizations—issued dire warnings about the future of nursing. The RWJ report, titled *Health Care's Human Crisis: The American Nursing Shortage*, underscored the need to "act soon" to "reverse the tide of what will become, if left unaddressed, a major public health crisis." In its 2002 report *Health Care at the Crossroads*, the Joint Commission described "a bad situation [that] only threatens to worsen. . . . [I]t is estimated that by 2020, there will be at least 400,000 fewer nurses available to provide care than will be needed." As a result, the Joint Commission cautioned, "the impending crisis in nurse staffing has the potential to impact the very health and security of our society if definitive steps are not taken to address its underlying causes."[19]

Although estimates of the magnitude of the staffing shortage varied, all shared a common theme: the problem was severe and rapidly worsening. The recitation of scary trends dominated media coverage of the nursing shortage. As CNN informed viewers in 2001, "The nursing shortage may be even worse than the medical community expected. Government figures show by the year 2008 an additional 450,000 nurses may be needed." In 2002 *Business Week* declared nursing was "on the critical list" and warned that "an acute shortage of RNs threatens to cripple U.S. hospitals."[20] Televised news reports painted a grim picture of the future of hospitals forced to curtail services and patients at risk because of a shortage of caregivers.

Each year brought more bad news. In 2003 *NBC News* noted that as a result of the "serious shortage of nurses in this country . . . more than a million new nurses will be needed by the year 2010. And if the profession continues on the track it's been on for the past several years, this goal will not be

met." That same year audiences learned that "America faces a nursing shortage of epidemic proportions." The future looked bleaker still, for news reports
noted that "the pipeline for future nurses is also dwindling." Once again, fear
framed debates over the nursing shortage, as reformers painted a desperate
picture of a future without caregivers. Fear-based appeals were commonplace in media coverage in recent years. As the *New York Times* asked, "Who's
going to take care of me someday? When I get old, when I get sick, who's
going to be there at my bedside?"[21]

An acute, and worsening, shortage of nurses represented an alarming
development in an aging society. The most recent nursing shortage came
at a time when millions of baby boomers were approaching retirement age.
Nurses argued that "we're only postponing the disaster that's going to happen eventually. There will not be enough nurses to care for us when all of
us reach the age where we need nursing care." Apocalyptic predictions of a
health care system without caregivers described a shrinking pool of nurses
struggling to care for millions of aging and disabled baby boomers. As the
New York Times editorialized in 2006, "The medical needs of an aging population make the nursing situation seem particularly stark. With the coming retirement of the last generation of women who chose nursing simply
because they didn't want to teach, things are likely to get only worse."[22]

Patients at Risk

A different narrative portrayed the shortage as a threat to the quality of
patient care. Nurses warned that the staffing crisis in hospitals placed
patients at risk. Inadequate staffing forced nurses to ration their time and
attention to the sickest patients, leaving others to fend for themselves. The
result was substandard, if not dangerous, care for many hospitalized patients.
By the early 1950s, hospital executives argued that "the prospect before us is
frightening. It cannot be denied that there are patients who suffer needlessly
and their recovery is retarded because of the critical nurse shortages. Our
most desperate plight is revealed during the afternoon and night shifts when
one nurse may have to assume responsibility for 400 to 600 patients." This
story of decline portrayed even elective surgeries or minor hospitalizations
as a threat to patient safety. Reporters warned that the "persistent shortage
of nurses has become so critical in New York City's municipal hospitals that
even routine nursing care is now largely reserved for the sickest patients
while healthier ones are left to take care of themselves."[23] The nursing shortage, under these circumstances, affected all patients. As stressed-out nurses

struggled to care for their sickest patients, they had little time to comfort and care for less acute cases.

Fears of preventable injuries or even deaths defined this narrative. Images of short-staffed hospitals shaped public perceptions, transforming treatment for common problems into a risky proposition. Such stories of the declining quality of patient care were commonplace in discussions of the nursing crisis over the past five decades. Each nursing shortage highlighted the same underlying threat to the quality of care: too many patients, too few nurses. By 2001 Americans learned that the "shortage of nurses and other health care workers represents a major health care crisis." In an environment defined by chronic understaffing, nurses were more prone to commit preventable, yet often deadly, errors. The net result of nursing vacancies "is longer hours and less time to carefully monitor patients." Television news reports warned that "far more effort is needed to ease a crisis that puts patients' lives at risk" in understaffed hospitals.[24] Nurses represent an "early warning system" for hospitalized patients. By carefully monitoring patient vital signs, observing patient behavior, and interacting with families at the bedside, nurses can avert potentially life-threatening infections or identify patients at risk.

Stories of tragic medical errors drew new attention to the nursing shortage. By the mid-1970s, news reports of deaths from medication errors due to overworked nurses attracted widespread public attention. In the wake of ongoing quality problems, physicians complained that at some New York hospitals, "a situation exists for the patient where it is more dangerous and life-threatening to come to the hospital than to stay at home." Nurses painted a grim picture of daily life in American hospitals. In 1981 nurses described being forced to "double up and work nonstop during their shifts and then frequently were asked to work overtime afterwards." As a result, one nurse at Lincoln Hospital noted that "when I begin my shift, I find out who is the sickest patient, and I decide that's who's going to get cared for. Now you may have other patients who do not get bathed when they should or get any exercise, or get any bedside attention." In this story, the shortage of nurses represented an imminent threat to patients. As *ABC News* informed viewers in 1981, "4 of 5 nurses in a national survey say they are unable to provide an acceptable level of care because of under-staffing, a condition reported by 60% of U.S. Hospitals." Stories of overworked nurses working extra shifts or caring for more patients during each shift underscored concerns about patient safety. *Business Week,* for example, described an obstetric nurse who "has so many patients in the maternity ward to look after that she often doesn't immediately notice when a fetal heart rate has slowed or an expectant mother has requested more pain medication."[25]

As one nurse wrote in the *New York Times*, "As a hospital patient, you have a right to qualified, alert, and dedicated nurses and other caregivers at your bedside. But these days you may be cared for by a nurse working her 16th hour, looking after 10 or more patients at a time. . . . If you are one of the patients waiting for help, you should also be concerned. Exhausted, stressed nurses can't provide the quality of care you deserve." The problem, as one ER nurse wrote in *Newsweek*, was simple: "too many patients, not enough staff. When I started emergency room nursing five years ago, I would typically have four or five patients . . . but now, on an average day, I have 10 to 12 patients. Once I even had 22. . . . Now, here's a question: do you want to be one of the five sickest who gets attention right away, or one of the others who have to wait maybe seven, eight, or even 10 hours before someone gets to you?" Nurses described a state of constant stress. As one nurse wrote in the *Wall Street Journal*, "I operated in a state of continuous low grade panic, punctuated by spikes of abject terror. The three or four nights a week when I walked toward the hospital to start my shift, I was gripped with a fear-induced nausea. My breathing quickened. Sweat slicked my palms. Please, don't let me hurt anyone tonight. Please."[26]

The flurry of stories about the medical consequences of understaffed hospitals was accompanied by ominous warnings for the public. News reports warned viewers, "There really is a crisis out there. People should be frightened. It is dangerous to be a patient." Stories noted that "inadequate nursing care can cause devastating problems for patients," as patients were more likely to suffer "serious complications, such as urinary tract infections, bleeding, and even death." As *NBC News* noted in 2002, "Inadequate staffing may contribute to nearly a quarter of hospital accidents that kill or injure patients." Horror stories portrayed the deadly consequences of the nursing shortage. *NBC Nightly News* described the plight of a Kansas woman whose mother "was flailing in bed, unable to breathe." Her daughter was "repeatedly pushing this call button for nobody to come." After actor Dennis Quaid's infant twins narrowly survived a near-fatal medication mix-up, viewers of *Today*—the nation's most watched morning newscast—learned about the role of understaffing in medical errors. As NBC's medical correspondent declared, "We have to stop getting by with the fact that we can understaff our hospitals with nurses and think it's OK. I think we have a phenomenal nursing shortage in this country, so shortcuts happen on the floor."[27]

Faced with potentially dangerous hospital stays, media reports underscored the need for patients to protect themselves. Anxious parents described bedside vigils caring for sick children in the hospital, as nurses were simply too busy with other patients to attend to them. A cottage industry of "how-to" stories appeared on television, online, and in bookstores, providing self-help tips for prospective patients. "To avoid becoming a victim of the nursing shortage," news reports advised viewers to "educate yourself and become your own best advocate." The result was a grim picture of a typical hospital stay. In an interview on CNN, Charles Inlander, the author of a "self-defense handbook for hospital patients," likened a hospital stay to "being a vacationing traveler who unknowingly wanders across a border into a combat zone where all the natives have guns at the ready." Vigilance was essential. "The whole issue with the nursing shortage is so critical because . . . the key care in the hospital is nursing care. It's not doctor care. You get virtually no care from your doctor at the hospital."[28] Patients, in short, needed to defend themselves in a hostile environment.

The Path Not Taken

To date, narratives of crisis have failed to mobilize public support for significant investments in nursing education and training opportunities. Federal leadership to address the nursing shortage through scholarships, faculty development, and the construction and expansion of nursing programs pales in comparison to support for graduate medical education. Crisis talk may actually exacerbate the shortage by dampening enthusiasm for the profession among potential nursing students. Images and stories of burned-out, stressed, and overworked nurses did little to increase the appeal of nursing relative to other health professions.

Horror stories about substandard care may fan public anxieties, but their power to mobilize Americans for political action depends upon individual circumstances. Most Americans also continue to express high levels of satisfaction with their recent encounters with health providers; for better or worse, most nurses have insulated their patients from the stresses of their daily work.[29] As a result, crisis language offers a poor description of most patients' interactions with nurses in hospital settings. This disconnection between lived experiences and crisis rhetoric undermines the credibility of such narratives and, in the process, drains the symbolic power of crisis as a catalyst for change.

More important, nurses and other advocates for reform misuse the concept of crisis to describe what is ultimately a chronic condition. Talk of a "persistent nursing shortage" dates back to the 1950s, when the *New York Times* reported that the nurse shortage was "serious" and "getting worse" across the United States. By the late 1950s, competition among hospitals to hire nurses resembled "something close to a frenzy." The 1960s brought no relief, as news reports described the shortage of nurses as "monumental" and "chronic."[30] As a chronic condition, the shortage of nurses requires careful monitoring, long-term treatment, and ongoing support, not episodic attention from policy makers and the press.

The nursing shortage is an example of a "dynamic shortage." Describing the shortage of engineers and scientists in the 1950s, Kenneth Arrow and William Capron note that persistent shortages can occur over time in markets where demand for workers continues to increase. Thus, even though the nursing supply grew steadily in the late twentieth century, the demand for nurses in hospitals, nursing homes, and outpatient settings outstripped the available supply. Since the demand for nurses continued to rise faster than the available supply, the market remained in a state of disequilibrium.[31]

By focusing on crisis stories, supporters of reform miss the opportunity to tell more powerful and credible narratives of progress. Nurses need to redefine public discourse to focus on their contributions to improving health outcomes. Reformers must engage patients, physicians, and third-party payers with a new narrative that focuses attention on patient safety. Such a story would engage the public with familiar themes of tragedy (preventable deaths), heroes (dedicated, well-trained nurses), and progress.

Just as Richard Nixon called on Americans to embrace "a total national commitment" to curing cancer, reformers must persuade policy makers and the public to embrace a new culture of patient safety. This new narrative has a simple, accessible message: high-quality nursing care, provided in well-staffed hospitals, saves lives. This new prescription would replace diagnoses of an emerging crisis with a call for safer hospitals and better care. This story is consistent with American beliefs in medical progress, for additional health care spending to cure disease and save lives has enjoyed widespread public support in the past.

A successful, long-term approach to reform must adopt a multipronged strategy to recruit and retain nurses in hospital settings. Although nurses focused increased attention on the need to prohibit mandatory overtime and institute minimum staffing ratios in recent years, neither approach addresses the principal cause of both: a shortage of nurses. Without additional nurses to meet the new demand, such regulations will simply ignite a bidding war among hospitals. The net result will exacerbate the shortage at already vulnerable institutions, shifting nurses from institutions with fewer resources to those who can afford to pay more. Staffing ratios and limitations on the use of mandatory overtime are important long-term goals to promote nurse retention and reduce burnout, but they cannot be implemented in isolation.

Instead, better funding for nursing education—and better working conditions for nurses—must be addressed as part of a long-term strategy to increase the nursing supply and enable hospitals to attract and retain nursing staff. With adequate staffing, hospitals could reduce the incidence and severity of medical errors. Recent studies of the relationship between nurse staffing and health care outcomes reinforce the importance of nurse staffing for patient outcomes. One study estimated that "if hospitals increased RN staffing and hours of nursing care per patient, more than 6,700 patient deaths and four million days of care in hospitals could be avoided each year."[32] From this perspective, America's failure to invest in the recruitment, training, and retention of nurses places patients at risk.

To address the chronic shortage of nurses, reformers must first focus on recruiting and retaining nursing faculty. In recent years, the shortage of qualified nursing faculty created a bottleneck at many of the nation's nursing schools; more than forty-two thousand qualified applicants were unable to enroll in nursing programs in 2006 due to a shortage of faculty.[33] The faculty shortage reflects current economic realities, as experienced nurses earn more working in hospital settings or as advanced practice nurses (that is, nurse practitioners, certified nurse midwives, or nurse anesthetists) than as faculty members. In this context, hiring new nursing faculty and increasing the capacity of nursing programs must be framed as investments in higher-quality, safer patient care.

Federal leadership is essential to address the nurse staffing shortfall. Recruitment—whether focused on faculty or students—must recognize that the nursing workforce is a public good. To attract more students to nursing, reformers must identify additional resources for scholarships and loan programs. States may, in certain cases, attract many students to inexpensive public nursing programs, but if a substantial proportion of program graduates leave to practice elsewhere, public support for state-level programs will be difficult to sustain. Indeed, despite the passage of the Nurse Reinvestment Act (Public Law 107-25) in 2002, federal funding for nursing education lags far behind that of graduate medical education. In the long run, federal support for nursing faculty and additional scholarships and loan-repayment programs is essential for increasing the affordability and appeal of nursing for prospective students.

The success of this new narrative, however, depends in large part on reshaping the image of the nursing profession. Nursing is often portrayed—either implicitly or explicitly—as less challenging, rewarding, and autonomous than careers in medicine or other allied health professions. Popular television shows such as *Chicago Hope, ER, Grey's Anatomy, House,* and *Royal Pains* are physician-centered medical dramas that present the daily life of physicians as one of constant challenge and excitement. In most medical dramas, nurses are typically cast in supporting roles, if they are featured at all. With few exceptions (for example, Carol Hathaway on *ER,* played by Julianna Margulies, and HBO's *Nurse Jackie,* played by Edie Falco), nurses on television medical dramas are marginal characters. The consequence of such casting decisions is significant, for "although real patients know that doctors do relatively little caregiving in hospitals, in the heroic medical narrative physicians do all of the curing and most of the caring. Non-physician caregivers are all but invisible in films and TV shows."[34] The real work of medicine —saving lives and healing patients—is performed by doctors on the most popular television medical dramas.

Since popular television programs serve as an important agent of socialization and reach millions of viewers each week, such portrayals are not inconsequential. Physician-centric dramas, according to critics, foster "long-standing misrepresentations that . . . are contributing to the nursing shortage. People think what they see on *ER* is real. Viewers, especially kids, see our profession as less than it really is, a horrible job. They see the show and think, 'Who would want to be a nurse?'" Such criticisms were not confined to *ER, Grey's Anatomy,* and "real-life" shows such as *Hopkins 24/7.* As Senator Barbara Mikulski (D-MD) observed, "ABC did not think that nursing was important" in casting *Hopkins 24/7,* for not one nurse was featured in the show.[35]

Popular sitcoms such as *Scrubs* also reinforced prevailing perceptions of nurses as "junior partners" in patient care. Although the *Scrubs* cast featured a strong female lead—nurse Carla Espinoza played a key role in teaching the new interns hands-on patient care—nurses enjoyed little professional autonomy at Sacred Heart Hospital. In the episode "My First Step," Espinoza's boyfriend and coworker, Dr. Chris Turk, encouraged her to return to school to become a nurse practitioner so she could "learn to how to be more than just a nurse." When Carla expressed frustration at Turk's lack of respect for her profession, Turk stood by his offer, noting that as an NP, "you'll have more responsibility and you'll make more money." Later in the same episode, the hospital's chief of medicine, Dr. Robert Kelso, lectured Carla for adjusting a patient's intravenous dosage. An indignant Kelso observed that "somebody went ahead and increased Mr. Brooks' lidocaine drip, and by law that could only be a doctor. Are you a doctor, Nurse Espinoza?"

By redefining public discourse about the nursing shortage in terms of patient protection, not an emerging crisis, policy makers can build upon public support for medical progress and the favorable image of the nursing profession. Efforts to remake the public image of nurses date back to the 1940s. Beginning in 1949, Chicago sought to raise awareness about the nursing shortage and improve the public image of nurses by creating a "Nurses' Day" and hosting an annual Chicago Nurse Parade. The city's treasurer argued that the "city and state should do everything possible to encourage young people to go into the nursing field and at the same time everything practical should be done to make the pay and working conditions of the nurse more attractive."[36] Similar efforts to change the public image of nursing as a profession were proposed during each nursing shortage in recent decades.

In recent years, initiatives such as Johnson and Johnson's Campaign for Nursing's Future produced a variety of recruitment materials such as brochures, pins, and posters for distribution to secondary schools. The company also sponsored a national advertising campaign using both print and online materials in an effort to "enhance the image of the nursing profession, recruit new nurses and nurse educators, and to retain nurses currently in the system." Although such private initiatives represent a promising beginning, the campaign's thirty-million-dollar budget was too small to reshape the image of the nursing profession. Although the campaign generated substantial private support for nursing scholarships and faculty development, fewer than one thousand student scholarships were awarded in the program's first three years.

To effect real change in public attitudes, "the community, media, government, church, business, and health care organizations need to unite with nurses to creatively address the importance and image of nurses. Continuous education and visibility are needed to describe the values and service of nurses, thus attracting more to enter the profession." The power of television to transform public attitudes about medical careers should not be underestimated. Interest in emergency medicine, in particular, increased substantially after the debut of *ER* in 1994.[37] Nurses must take a page from physicians' playbook, for doctors have worked closely with Hollywood for decades to create popular medical dramas that highlight the contributions of doctors for millions of television viewers. Public service announcements, while useful, must be seen as part of an overall media strategy that includes efforts to redefine the role of nurses. If popular shows such as *Grey's Anatomy* and *House* focused attention on nurses' role in preventing medical errors, resuscitating patients, or monitoring the health of critically ill patients, audiences would gain a fuller understanding of the range, and autonomy, of nursing practice.

The use of crisis narratives to describe the continued shortage of nurses offers a vivid example of how language hinders our understanding of policy problems. The nursing shortage is ultimately a long-term, chronic challenge for the American health care system. Crisis talk has done little to rally public support for long-term investments in nursing education, training, or improved working conditions. Instead of fearmongering, reformers must tell a new story that captures the public imagination and celebrates the vital importance of nursing as a profession for future generations.

CHAPTER FIVE

The Health Insurance Crisis

By any reasonable definition, there is a crisis in insurance coverage when tens of millions of Americans remain uninsured and live in constant fear of bankruptcy should they become ill.   —"Yes, There Is a Health Crisis," editorial, *New York Times*, January 30, 1994

There are an estimated 46 million Americans who don't have health insurance. . . . This is a national health care crisis.
                —Peter Jennings, "Breakdown: America's Health Insurance Crisis," *Prime Time Live*, December 15, 2005

SINCE THE EARLY 1970s, advocates of national health insurance framed debates over universal coverage using the language and imagery of crisis. A familiar cycle emerged during each reform period, as elected officials and interest groups raised warnings of an emerging crisis in the nation's health insurance system. Reformers argued that the impending implosion of the nation's health insurance system demanded immediate action, and public officials and the mass media hailed the passage of reform as "inevitable." Opponents, however, succeeded in redefining the terms of public discourse each time national health insurance appeared on the policy agenda. Ideological foes and affected interest groups defined reformers' prescription for the uninsured—universal coverage—as worse than the disease itself.

Crisis narratives appeared in a variety of different settings, including political campaigns, legislative debates, news coverage, popular magazines, and televised documentaries. The narrators of this story varied, and included political candidates, interest-group representatives, reporters, and even characters in popular television programs and movies. Each narrative of crisis varied, but all reinforced the sense that the system was rapidly deteriorating. The principal protagonists in these stories of crisis were hardworking families facing circumstances beyond their control.

Similar arguments reappeared during the contentious debates over health care reform in 2009–10. Ironically, the passage of the Patient Protection and Affordable Care Act (Public Law 111-148) illustrated the dysfunctional character of public discourse about health care reform. Within a year of its passage, the fragile consensus in support of universal coverage began to fray. The PPACA was also the first major social reform to be enacted by Congress on a party-line vote, without a single Republican vote in either chamber. Ironically, the principal beneficiaries of the new law were Republican challengers and Democratic legislators who cast votes against the bill.

Public disillusionment with health care reform contributed to the "shellacking" suffered by President Obama and congressional Democrats in the 2010 midterm elections. During the fall campaign, Democratic candidates distanced themselves from the bill, or sought to explain their votes to a skeptical electorate. Remarkably, more Americans believed that their families would be worse off after the passage of reform than felt they would benefit from the new law. Less than a year after the passage of the PPACA, a plurality of Americans (46 percent) favored its repeal. Reformers, in short, had failed to weave a persuasive policy story for voters. By January 2011, more members of the House cast votes to repeal the PPACA (245) than had supported it (219) less than ten months earlier, and twenty-seven states banded together to challenge the constitutionality of the new law in federal courts. The result, as Atul Gawande has observed, is that "the battle for health-care reform has only begun."[1]

This ongoing stalemate has its roots in the language of health care reform and, in particular, in the narratives of crisis used to frame public debates about the need for universal coverage. Supporters of the new law—including President Obama and congressional Democrats—blamed "misleading" attacks and a "stunningly effective misinformation campaign" waged by Republicans for stoking public opposition. As President Obama noted in his address to Congress in September 2009, "Given all the misinformation that's been spread over the past few months, I realize that many Americans have grown nervous about reform." Media analyses denounced the "lies and fantasies about health care reform" and dismissed attacks on the new law as a "sort of lunatic paranoia—touched with populism, nativism, racism, and anti-intellectualism [that] has long been a feature of the fringe, especially during times of economic bewilderment." Surveying the continued controversy over health care reform after the passage of the PPACA, academic observers attributed public hostility to reform to "the legacy of 'death panels,' a 'government takeover of health care,' and other incendiary—but false and misleading—charges made by the law's opponents."[2]

Complaints about the quality of public deliberation in health care reform are not new and are reminiscent of the raucous ideological battles over "socialized medicine" and Medicare from the 1940s to the 1960s. Such complaints, however, miss a larger point. Storytelling is vital to the future of health insurance reform in America. In 1990 Health and Human Services secretary Louis Sullivan said, "There is no consensus in this country on how to achieve the kind of health care system we want, or how the cost of improvements in our health care system should be borne."[3] Two decades later, Sullivan's observation still rings true. Unless and until reformers address this basic task of building public support for universal coverage, health insurance reforms will continue to rest on a shaky foundation.

Nearly four decades after Richard Nixon first warned Americans of an emerging crisis in the nation's health insurance system, crisis narratives have been repeated so often, and in so many different settings, that they are now firmly embedded in popular culture and politics. Such rhetoric, however, offers a vivid example of "language on holiday," for the dire depictions of a crumbling health care system do not resemble the experiences of most Americans—85 percent of whom are covered by either public or private health insurance. For insured Americans, "day-to-day access to the health care system may be somewhat confusing, inconvenient, or unpredictable, but it does not seem by any means intolerable."[4] Despite repeated cries of crisis, insured patients continue to express high levels of satisfaction with their own coverage and access to providers.

Crisis talk raises many questions that are often unasked, and therefore unanswered, by reformers. For example, what does it mean to say that the health insurance system in the United States is in a state of crisis? How is the crisis defined? What, if anything, will happen in the absence of reform? Furthermore, why have repeated warnings of an emerging crisis failed to generate a broad-based social movement to press for universal coverage?

Narratives of Crisis

Beginning in 1969, supporters of health care reform redefined public debate about universal coverage using the rhetoric of crisis. Their rhetoric displayed a remarkable consistency over time, even as the nature of policy proposals changed substantially; the same symbolic stories and images reappeared each time universal health insurance returned to the public agenda. Proponents of universal health insurance employed several familiar narratives to mobilize public support for national health insurance in recent decades. Each was bound together by a common thread of fear. These stories and

symbols reinforced the urgency of reform by describing a health insurance
system that was on the brink of collapse. Without swift action to control
spiraling insurance premiums, both policy makers and the media argued
that millions of working- and middle-class families would soon find private
health insurance unaffordable.

Opponents of national health insurance also used fear to frame public
debates over national health insurance. By appealing to Americans' traditional fears of "big government" and their distrust of bureaucracy, opponents of national health insurance redefined the terms of political discourse.
Rather than focusing on the need for universal coverage, opponents warned
of a new crisis that revolved around the scope of government involvement
in the health care system and the larger economy. Doctors, insurers, and
business groups warned that government-sponsored health insurance was
inconsistent with basic American values and represented a fundamental
shift in the role of the federal government. National health insurance, unlike
existing public health insurance programs such as Medicare and Medicaid
that targeted benefits to the elderly and poor, had the potential to affect virtually every American. This narrative also tapped into deep-rooted public
concerns about "big government" to undermine public support for reform.
Rather than solving the nation's health care problems, critics argued that a
system of national health insurance would decrease patient choice, erode the
quality of patient care, and create a tangle of bureaucratic red tape. Passage
of reform, in this policy story, would plunge the health care system—which
worked well for most Americans—into chaos, undermining confidence in
both government and health care institutions.

Similar to Grant McConnell's description of the "orthodox" and "progressive" traditions in American society, these two policy narratives coexisted
uneasily during each debate over health insurance reform from the early
twentieth century to the present day. Each has roots in deep-seated political
and social values.

Constructing the Health Insurance Crisis

For most of the twentieth century, efforts to enact national health insurance
in America were typically defined in terms of social progress. Significantly,
polls found little dissatisfaction with the overall state of the health care system. Neither policy makers nor the public framed the need for health care
reform as a crisis. In 1969, however, President Richard Nixon warned that the
"nation is faced with a breakdown in the delivery of health care unless imme-

diate concerted action is taken by Government and the private sector." Spear-
headed by the efforts of Walter Reuther, the president of the United Auto
Workers, a broad-based Committee for National Health Insurance pressed
for a "complete reshaping" of the American health care system. The committee—which included Senator Edward M. Kennedy (D-MA), noted philan-
thropist Mary Lasker, and pioneering heart surgeon Dr. Michael DeBakey—
lobbied for a "uniquely American" system of national health insurance.[5]

Without fundamental reform, advocates of national health insurance
argued that millions of Americans would be denied care, or risk financial ruin
to pay for it. As Senator Edward M. Kennedy declared in 1971, "The American
health care system is in crisis, and this crisis is deepening. The reality of this
crisis, which affects almost every citizen, is no longer denied." The precise
nature and meaning of the crisis, however, remained up for grabs. Few policy
makers felt a need to define the essence of the health insurance crisis, and
fewer still questioned the underlying premise that the system was poised on
the verge of collapse. As Roger Egeberg declared in 1970, "The signs of the
health care crisis are obvious and predictable." A quarter century later, Governor Robert Casey (D-PA) sounded a similar theme, arguing, "We all know
it's a crisis. It's been diagnosed to death. It's time long past to stop pointing
with alarm at the problem and start doing something about it."[6]

As the number of uninsured Americans increased from 31 million in
1987 to more than 38 million in 1992, health care reform emerged as a domi-
nant issue in both the 1988 and the 1992 presidential campaigns. By 1991
the *Journal of the American Medical Association*—one of the nation's leading academic medical journals—editorialized that the health care system
was "poised on the verge of a . . . meltdown." As Senator Edward Kennedy
declared in 1992, "Every family that is watching your program this morning
has seen a dramatic increase in terms of hospital bills, doctors' bills, premiums that they pay on health insurance. Every family here knows that there's
a real crisis in America."[7] Such dire warnings dramatized the need for urgent
action to repair the nation's health insurance system.

Images of the uninsured in popular culture humanized the health insurance crisis for the public. Popular television shows such as *ER, Grey's Anatomy,* and *Royal Pains* dramatized the personal struggles uninsured families
faced. Films that highlighted the shortcomings of the American health insurance industry such as *The Rainmaker, As Good as It Gets,* and *John Q* also
grossed millions at the box office. In theaters, moviegoers shouted at the

screen and applauded as characters vented their frustration with the rising cost of health care and the behavior of health insurers.

The first season of ABC's blockbuster drama *Grey's Anatomy*, for example, introduced viewers to the painful choices that the uninsured faced. Meredith Grey and her colleagues regularly socialized after work at a local bar, whose good-natured owner, Joe, befriended many of the physicians and residents from nearby Seattle Grace Hospital. In the episode "Raindrops Keep Falling on My Head," Joe begged the assembled doctors to not bring him to the hospital after he collapsed at work because he had no health insurance. Despite his protests, the doctors brought Joe to Seattle Grace Hospital anyway, where tests revealed that he had an aneurysm in his brain. This episode brought the fundamental insecurity the uninsured face home to millions of viewers. For the uninsured, cost is not only an issue, but *the* issue. As Joe noted, "I own a bar, and I don't got any insurance, so I'm not that concerned about the surgery as what I'm gonna do when I survive it." Joe's principal concern was not about the outcome of his surgery or its risks, but rather the cost of his care. This fear—the awareness that lifesaving care exists, but may be beyond reach—is an enduring theme in the rhetoric of crisis that has framed public discussion of health insurance reform in America.

By personalizing the plight of the uninsured, narratives of crisis portray the uninsured as familiar, not strange. Heart-wrenching profiles of uninsured patients struggling to obtain needed care and of families burdened by the rising cost of health insurance featured prominently in news coverage, political campaigns, and popular culture. Joe, for example, was a hardworking, affable character. The use of a middle-class owner of a small business as the face of the uninsured in this episode normalized the plight of the uninsured for the audience. Joe, in short, was Everyman. As a small businessman, he simply could not afford coverage. Through Joe, millions of viewers met the uninsured, and they are us. The fear of financial ruin uninsured families face is a defining feature of policy narratives about the crisis of health insurance. Stories of patients being denied care, hospitals teetering on the brink of bankruptcy, and families living in constant fear of illness frame public understanding of both the shortcomings of the health care system and the range of potential solutions. The lack of health insurance, in short, was a matter of life and death in the cries of crisis that defined public debate over health care reform.

Crisis rhetoric crossed party lines, and the extent to which members of

both parties accepted the prevailing notion of an emerging crisis is remarkable. Leaders as diverse as Richard Nixon, Jimmy Carter, John McCain, and
Barack Obama all endorsed the notion of a health insurance crisis. Senator
Hillary Clinton (D-NY) summarized this diagnosis on the campaign trail,
declaring that "our health care system . . . is, simply put, broken." Clinton's
sentiments were mirrored by one of the principal critics of the health care
reform bill in 2010, Senator Judd Gregg (R-NH), who wrote that "everyone
agrees that the health care system in this country is broken."[8]

The debate over health care reform in the 2008 presidential campaign
resembled previous debates over national health insurance in the 1970s and
1990s. Each of the leading contenders for the presidency in 2008—Hillary
Clinton, John Edwards, John McCain, and Barack Obama—offered their own
plans for reform, and all endorsed the notion that the American health insurance system faced a crisis. Too many Americans, McCain noted, "don't have
any insurance policy at all, and those who do are afraid they will lose the one
they have—afraid they will get too sick, afraid to stay home and not work
full time, and afraid that their benefits will disappear along with their job."[9]
In this story, the erosion of the health insurance system was a direct, not an
indirect, threat for insured Americans.

Reformers argued that the worsening condition of the American health
insurance system demanded immediate attention from policy makers. The
language of crisis that policy makers and the press used fanned public fears
that the health insurance system was in disarray. Even Karl Rove—a leading
domestic policy adviser for President George W. Bush—noted in 2007 that
"all around America, families are grappling with health care concerns. They
wonder if they'll have insurance at a price they can afford. They worry about
how much out-of-pocket costs take from the family budget. They question if
they'll be able to pick their own doctor. Some feel trapped in jobs they don't
like out of fear of losing health insurance." Similarly, Hendrick Hertzberg
wrote in the *New Yorker,* "Our health care system continues to deteriorate.
. . . Thirty-eight million Americans were uninsured in 2000; now it's forty-
seven million. Employer based health insurance is increasingly expensive,
stingy, and iffy."[10] The words used to describe the crisis varied—*breakdown,
catastrophe, collapse, meltdown*—but each evoked the language and imagery
of fear.

Crisis narratives from the 1970s to the present day featured three distinct
stories of decline. The first focused attention on the trials and tribulations
of Americans without health insurance as they struggled to obtain care. The

characters in this story were ordinary Americans who faced extraordinary financial hardships because they lacked health insurance. The uninsured, in this narrative, were victims of circumstances beyond their control. In an employer-based health insurance system, Americans who lost a job, or switched to a new job, risked losing their insurance coverage. Using a simple story of control, reformers asked the public to imagine a future where national health insurance provided affordable care to all and insulated all Americans from financial ruin.

The second story of decline described desperate families who were denied needed care because they could not afford it. This narrative highlighted heart-wrenching profiles of patients who were unable to pay for vital services. In particular, news reports personalized the health insurance crisis for the public by presenting the "human face" behind the statistics. For millions of Americans, universal coverage was a matter of life and death.

A third—and related—story of decline described the broadening reach of the health insurance crisis. In this narrative, spiraling premiums threatened the ability of millions of insured Americans to maintain their coverage. Political candidates and the media focused attention on the impact of rising insurance premiums on family budgets. Stories of decline portrayed health insurance premiums as a millstone around the neck of working- and middle-class families. Once again, "average families" served as the public face of the health insurance crisis for policy makers and the public. Responsibility for the crisis in the nation's health insurance system was placed at the feet of insurers, employers, and, in many cases, health providers.

Crisis narratives from the 1970s to the present day used fears of financial ruin to describe the economic impact of limited health insurance coverage— or the lack of it altogether—on average Americans. Writing in the *Atlantic Monthly* in 1970, Michael Crichton captured public anxieties with his description of John O'Connor, a middle-class patient whose expenses for one month in a hospital intensive care unit exceeded his annual salary. O'Connor's seventeen-foot-long hospital bill dramatized public fears that even one episode of illness could wipe out a family's savings. This lurking fear of bankruptcy—or unaffordable levels of debt to pay for needed care—is commonplace in public discourse about the health insurance crisis. As Harry Schwartz noted in 1970, "In these days of rising medical costs, a recurrent nightmare of millions of middle class families is the specter of financial ruin caused by catastrophic illness." Narratives of crisis emphasized both the breadth of the financial threat and its seemingly random nature. Policy makers stoked public anxieties about the growing incidence of the crisis and its impact on the uninsured. Senator Edward Kennedy wrote in 1972, "Families which are torn by illness have been forced to sell their homes, to sacrifice in a few weeks savings accumulated over years of hard work, to move in with relatives, and to live in near poverty—all to pay the costs of their tragic illness or accident."[11] Unanticipated illness or injury struck without warning, devastating the best-laid plans of hardworking Americans.

Two decades later, *CBS News* described a health care system in critical condition. "People are going bankrupt. They're losing their houses. They can't afford to get their kids through college anymore. They're just struggling to either pay the amount of money that they have to spend on medical care or making other choices that are very serious—losing their homes. This is a crisis that has to be dealt with." The fear of unaffordable health care costs also defined much of the public discourse over health care reform in the early 1990s, as public opinion polls revealed that more than a third of the public worried about paying for medical or health costs.[12]

The politics of fear was also central to the public debate over health insurance reform during the Clinton administration. The essence of the health insurance crisis, Clinton argued, was that "millions of Americans are just a pink slip away from losing their health insurance, and one serious illness away from losing all of their savings." This story of decline framed the president's nationally televised address to Congress in September 1993. Clinton declared that the health insurance crisis was evident in "the for-sale signs in front of the homes of families who've lost everything because of health care costs." The public image of the uninsured underscored the legitimacy of their appeal for government action. In sharp contrast to public debates about welfare reform in the 1980s and 1990s that often castigated the poor as "welfare queens" or "cheats," news reports portrayed the uninsured as victims of circumstances beyond their control. In contrast, crisis narratives absolved the uninsured for their predicament. As the US Senate began its floor debate over health care reform in 1994, Senator George Mitchell (D-ME) decried the fact that "high costs are driving ordinary Americans to choices that no civilized society should tolerate. Why is our society willing to allow people to experience the degradation, the humiliation of begging for care after a lifetime of hard work and personal responsibility? It's not fair. It should not continue. There are too many people forced into this kind of choice."[13]

Horror stories of Americans devastated by unexpected health care costs underscored the proximity of the crisis for all families. During the 1992 vice presidential debate, for example, Senator Al Gore (D-TN) described the experience of "a friend of mine named Mitch Philpott . . . who Tipper and I met with his family in Johns Hopkins Hospital. Their son Brett was in the bed next to our son, and they couldn't pay their medical bills. They used to live in Atlanta, but they lost their house."[14]

President Clinton echoed this story when he described the plight of the Anderson family in his 1994 State of the Union address: "Richard Anderson . . . lost his job and with it, his health insurance. Two weeks later his wife, Judy, suffered a cerebral aneurysm. He rushed her to the hospital, where she stayed in intensive care for 21 days. The Andersons' bills were over $120,000. Although Judy recovered and Richard went back to work at $8 an hour, the bills were too much for them and they were literally forced into bankruptcy. . . . I know there are people here who say there's no health care crisis. Tell it to Richard and Judy Anderson."[15] By sharing these stories with the public, political candidates and policy makers personalized the health insurance crisis and underscored the arbitrary and capricious nature of catastrophic health care costs. Families such as the Andersons and the Philpotts were innocent victims of the health insurance crisis, for no one could anticipate the need for such expensive, lifesaving medical procedures.

Familiar narratives of decline reappeared when health insurance reform returned to the public agenda during the 2008 presidential campaign. The AMA's Voice for the Uninsured campaign underscored the proximity of health insurance reform. The forty-seven million uninsured, they noted, were "not just a number or graph in a report. It's people all around you. Like a friend. A neighbor. A relative. People who are suffering."[16]

Contenders for the presidency from both parties warned voters that unforeseen circumstances could place them at risk of bankruptcy. As Senator Hillary Rodham Clinton told voters in 2007, "The devastation when one stroke of bad luck undoes a lifetime of hard work" provided ample evidence of a crisis in the nation's health insurance system. Campaigning in Iowa, Senator Barack Obama (D-IL) related stories of small business owners driven into bankruptcy by uncovered medical bills. Obama argued, "We have reached a point in this country where the rising cost of health care has put too many families and businesses on a collision course with financial ruin and left too many without coverage at all." The health insurance crisis had bipartisan appeal as a campaign issue in 2008. As Senator John McCain

(R-AZ) warned voters in 2007, "We are approaching a 'perfect storm' of problems, that if not addressed by the next president, will cause our health care system to implode."[17]

News coverage of the uninsured also displayed a remarkable continuity over time. In 1994, for example, the *New York Times* chided critics of the Clinton plan who "do not see a crisis . . . when 60 million Americans a year face the fear of bankruptcy from medical catastrophe." By 2007 *U.S. News and World Report* noted that "tens of millions of Americans live in fear that a major health problem can reduce them to bankruptcy. They realize their families are one health crisis away from family hardship, which is a key reason for the pervasive feeling of personal and permanent insecurity."[18]

Horror stories featured prominently in media coverage of health care reform. Television newscasts and documentaries described the struggles of families burdened with overwhelming and unanticipated health care costs. Charles Gibson, the cohost of *Good Morning America,* emphasized the common ground between insured and uninsured Americans in a 2003 segment. "The health care crisis," Gibson told viewers, "is really about you and me and all of our families. So many people [are] not covered by health care insurance. . . . We're going to begin our week-long [series] . . . with the story of an ordinary family that is facing, well, just ordinary health care bills, but it's driving them to bankruptcy." Images of hardworking families, sick children, and other visible victims of the health insurance crisis humanized the recitation of statistics about the number of uninsured Americans. Heart-wrenching human-interest profiles, such as the *CBS Early Show*'s story of an uninsured couple saddled with a $116,000 hospital bill, resembled Michael Crichton's vivid description of the cost of care a quarter century before. As Diane Sawyer warned viewers of *Good Morning America* in 2005, "Many Americans are just one serious illness away from financial catastrophe, bankruptcy." A year later, *Good Morning America* reported that "a record number of Americans are facing a frightening new life without health insurance," forcing some Americans to "choos[e] food over health coverage. . . . And it's only getting worse."[19] The implicit—or explicit—warning of such stories was that no one was safe from the threat of catastrophic health care costs.

The uninsured faced not only financial ruin, but also confronted lingering fears of death and disability. Crisis narratives also warned that Americans without health insurance coverage would be denied care. As Roger Egeberg, the assistant secretary of HEW, warned, "The 1970s will see the most severe test of America's capacity to deliver decent health care to those who need it.

. . . [M]illions of Americans simply are not getting needed health care."[20] The health insurance system, in this story, was a potentially fatal threat to the health of American families.

Senator Edward Kennedy's 1972 book, *In Critical Condition,* captured the awful dilemma the uninsured and underinsured faced: "When Americans who can pay little or nothing for care are struck by illness or accident, they have two choices. They can seek treatment from private hospitals and physicians at the risk of being turned away because they cannot pay or they can seek care from a city or charity hospital where care is frequently demeaning and inadequate. Unfortunately, many Americans avoid both alternatives. Rather than risk humiliation, they simply avoid taking members of their family for care at all, except in grave emergencies when they have no choice."[21]

This narrative featured prominently in the debate over health insurance reform during the early 1990s as well. In an employer-based system, joblessness could lead not only to economic ruin, but even death. In a televised address to the nation in September 1993, Clinton declared that "it is our turn to strike a blow for freedom in this country. The freedom of Americans to live without fear that their own nation's health care system won't be there for them when they need it." In considering proposals for health care reform, Clinton asked legislators to "look into the eyes of a sick child who needs care. To think of the face of a woman who has been told that her condition is malignant, but not covered by her insurance."[22]

Media reports warned of a growing problem as uninsured patients scrambled to obtain needed care. In 1983 the *New York Times* observed that "of all the pain and problems the recession has caused, none may be as severe or long-lasting as the damage done to the health of people who, having lost their medical insurance along with their jobs, are not getting the care they need." Soon after President Clinton's inauguration in 1993, *ABC News* reported, "Across the country today, health care is systematically being rationed. . . . It's a story the new President Bill Clinton can hear in almost any hospital in the country. . . . People cannot afford health insurance, and hospitals cannot afford to treat them."[23]

By 2007 news reports described desperate individuals "ready to go to Washington [themselves] if that would help get Congress to do something about the health insurance crisis that is responsible for so much unnecessary suffering and death in the U.S." As the *New York Times* noted, "Americans with inadequate health coverage—the underinsured—are a major component of the national health crisis. Like the uninsured, they can be denied desperately needed treatment for financial reasons; they often suffer financial ruin and in many cases they die unnecessarily." Writing in *Newsweek* in 2007, former vice presidential candidate Geraldine Ferraro (D-NY), a cancer survivor, declared that "I've seen firsthand just how broken our nation's health care system is. People who have insurance and money get the treatment they need to live, and those who don't—well, it's a crapshoot—it's unconscionable that we have a health care system where people are denied the treatment they need because they can't afford it."[24] Once again, the plight of uninsured Americans was portrayed not as a choice, but rather as a consequence of circumstances beyond their control. Stories of the uninsured emphasized that losing health insurance, or being uninsured, typically resulted from the decisions of employers, the consequences of foreign competition, or the state of the economy.

Television news coverage of the uninsured had a strong interpretive flavor. News anchors and reporters did not merely describe the problems facing uninsured families, but also shared their own values and opinions with viewers. In a 1991 segment on the *CBS Evening News,* anchor Dan Rather highlighted the scope of the crisis for viewers. Rather described the nation's health care system as a "national shame" and decried the fact that "in ours, the wealthiest nation on earth, millions of people cannot afford to go to the doctor." Rather's observations were reminiscent of Walter Cronkite's famous commentary on the prospects of winning the war in Vietnam. In this context, reporters not only described the number of Americans without health insurance, but also endorsed the need for universal coverage as a matter of shared risk. Access to health care in America, in short, had become a "matter of life and debt." News reports were replete with horror stories of the life-or-death stories facing uninsured patients. As *CBS News* reporter Edie Magnus told viewers, "For the millions of Americans who don't have health insurance, the prospect of illness or accidents can be paralyzing. . . . Americans share [a] sense of doom. Almost eight out of 10 surveyed think this country is heading for a health care crisis."[25] Vivid images of desperate families, preventable disease, and premature death highlighted the urgency of efforts to pass universal health insurance.

Stories of uninsured patients who were unable to obtain health care for chronic yet life-threatening problems were a common feature of media reports. Viewers of the *CBS Evening News,* for example, learned about the health insurance crisis through the eyes of Pearl Farrell in 1990. "Like 37 million other Americans, 80% of them employed, Pearl Farrell has no health insurance. She works in a small beauty salon that doesn't provide it." Ms. Farrell warned, "If anything was to happen major, I wouldn't be covered, and I would have a lot of problems paying my bill." A year later, *ABC News Nightline* repeated this theme in its profile of jobless Americans struggling to pay for care. "Like the millions who suddenly find themselves unemployed, Jack Stalter could not afford health insurance on his own, and without insurance, he could not afford the medicine he urgently needed." Stalter declared, "Because of lack of medication, I was having a lot of problems with hypertension—high blood pressure—along with angina and severe vascular headaches. I got so sick that I didn't care whether I lived or died." Similar profiles of desperate patients can be found throughout the debate over health care reform in the 1990s. In 1992 *ABC News* introduced viewers to Karen Allen, "one of an estimated 80 million Americans who are living on the edge, people who are in physical and financial jeopardy because either they do not have health insurance or they are in danger of losing it."[26] Profiles of Pearl, Jack, Karen, and other uninsured patients became the public face of the health insurance crisis. Through these testimonials, viewers who had not personally fallen through the cracks of the health insurance system learned about the consequences of being uninsured.

Reformers also warned that the current system of private health insurance coverage was increasingly insecure and warned insured Americans that they too might be at risk. The escalating cost of employer-sponsored insurance coverage threatened access to affordable health care for working families. As House Speaker Thomas Foley (D-WA) declared in 1992, "Today millions of Americans have no health insurance at all. And even those who do have no assurance that they are safe. People worry that if they get sick, their coverage will be canceled. Premiums and out of pocket costs continue to multiply. Workers who lose their jobs suddenly find their children with no insurance."[27] In this story of decline, everyone was at risk—insured and uninsured alike.

News stories underscored the threat of the eroding system of employer-based coverage for currently insured families. By the early 1990s, morning news shows warned viewers that "if you think health insurance is expensive now, get ready, because it's going to cost even more in the next few years." By 1991 the *New York Times* reported that "for the public, fear is growing." As *NBC News* anchor Tom Brokaw asked viewers in 1997, "Even if you've earned a pension, saved money, and worked out a budget for early retirement, can you be sure your health insurance will be there? If you're sure you'll be covered, you may want to think again." Two years later, Dan Rather described the "health care squeeze" to viewers of the *CBS Evening News*. Rather stoked viewers' latent anxieties about the deterioration of private health insurance coverage by asking viewers, "What if you have insurance? Are you sure you'll be covered if you get sick?"[28]

Media reports framed rapidly rising health insurance costs as a crisis for the middle class. Escalating costs threatened the financial well-being of insured families. As the *New York Times* observed in 2002, "The health care crisis is spreading up the income ladder and deep into the ranks of those with full time jobs." The implication of this worrisome trend was that fewer Americans would be able to depend on private, employer-sponsored coverage in the future. As one worker interviewed by the *New York Times* in 2002 quipped, "I don't know where it stops. With a 20 percent increase each year, over time the only two people in this country who will be able to have health insurance are Bill Gates and Warren Buffett. No one else can afford it." Even the language used to describe rising health insurance costs stoked public concerns, as media coverage warned viewers about "surging" premiums.[29]

This story of decline reinforced the proximity of health insurance reform for all Americans. In 2004 Katie Couric—the cohost of NBC's *Today*—introduced viewers to an uninsured man who was "afraid millions more Americans could soon be forced to live without insurance, just like he is." The segment ended with a grim warning about the expanding reach of the health insurance crisis: "If it's not affecting you, it will someday. It will someday." *ABC News* anchor Peter Jennings spent the last months of his life working on a documentary—*Breakdown*—about the health insurance crisis. His final project for *Primetime Live* introduced viewers to "America's health insurance crisis." The crisis, Jennings declared, "touches every American. . . . [Health insurance] is hard to get. It is hard to keep. And it is increasingly hard to afford."[30] Reformers cited continued increases in health insurance premiums and the declining number of businesses that offered coverage to their workers as evidence that the system was collapsing.

A Second Opinion

Each effort to enact a system of national health insurance, however, sparked intense opposition. For businesses, insurers, and physicians, reform represented a slippery slope of government intervention that raised the prospect of a different kind of crisis. Opponents viewed health care reform itself as the problem. In this alternative diagnosis, national health insurance would create a crisis of confidence in both the health care system and American political institutions. Critics celebrated private solutions to improve access to health care and derided national health insurance as a costly prescription for "big government." This policy story drew upon what James Morone describes as "vague but potent American traditions celebrating individualism, promoting market competition, and bashing governments."[31] The counternarratives offered by opponents defined publicly funded health insurance as a powerful symbolic enemy.

National health insurance, in this narrative, was inconsistent with American values. A second story of decline challenged the legitimacy of national health insurance. Universal coverage, critics argued, would simply lead to "big government." Images of faceless government bureaucracies became a powerful weapon for opponents of national health insurance each time reform appeared on the national policy agenda. Opponents of government-funded health insurance tapped into public preferences for limited government and voluntarism, rather than public regulation and taxation, as the preferred path to provide for the uninsured. Government, in short, was viewed as a threat to patient choice and personal liberty.

Opponents insisted that proposals for universal health insurance were unworkable or unaffordable. The "side effects" of national health insurance, in this policy narrative, would leave Americans with less freedom, poorer-quality medical care, and higher taxes. These arguments closely paralleled the theses of perversity, futility, and jeopardy described by Albert O. Hirschman in *The Rhetoric of Reaction*. "According to the perversity thesis, any purposive action to improve some features of the political, social, or economic order only serves to exacerbate the condition one wishes to remedy. The futility thesis holds that any attempts at social transformation will be unavailing, that they will simply fail to 'make a dent.' Finally, the jeopardy thesis argues that the cost of the proposed change or reform is too high as it endangers some previous, precious accomplishment." [32]

Fears of "big government" provided a powerful symbolic enemy for opponents of national health insurance over the past four decades. The result of such fears, Samuel Huntington observes, is that "political authority is vulnerable in America as it is nowhere else." As President Dwight Eisenhower argued in 1952, "Federal compulsion, with our health supervised under a Washington stethoscope, is not American and it is not the answer. Instead of more and better medical care it would give us poorer medical care." This lingering suspicion of government reflects the enduring relevance of what

Grant McConnell described as the orthodox tradition in American politics. Opponents of national health insurance repeatedly tapped the public's "deep-seated faith in the virtue of small units of political and social organization." Voluntary associations and private groups were celebrated by generations of candidates and interest groups. "By contrast, government, especially the national government, parties, and 'politics' in general have been deplored as threats to liberty."[33]

The notion of government as a symbolic enemy in public deliberations over health care reform dates back to the early twentieth century and has reappeared in each subsequent reform era. As Senator Orrin Hatch (R-UT) argued during committee hearings over a "play or pay" bill in 1992, "I have never heard of any product or service, which, if regulated by government, you get a better choice, quality, and supply." Two decades later, opponents of the Obama administration's proposals for health care reform raised similar concerns that questioned the ability of government to solve the health care system's problems. "Think of everything you know about public housing, the image the term conjures up in your mind. If you like public housing you will love public health care." Senator Chuck Grassley (R-IA) signaled his disapproval of Democratic proposals for health care reform in 2009, noting that "the reform proposals pending in Congress would make a bad situation worse. These bills would cause us to slide rapidly down the slippery slope toward increasing government control over health care. . . . A government run plan would eventually drive private insurers out of business and lead to a government takeover of the health care system."[34]

The enduring appeal of private solutions to public problems also resurfaced in each debate over national health insurance. As Anthony Lewis noted in 1976, campaigning against big government is an "old fashioned theme, but an entirely relevant one. . . . Americans of all kinds now feel, and resent, the heavy hand of Washington bureaucracy." Playing upon this fear of "big government," opponents branded proposals for national health insurance as a cure far worse than the disease. In the three decades since Lewis wrote those words, "running against Washington" became a bipartisan strategy. On the campaign trail, candidates routinely celebrated the virtues of private citizens and organizations and decried the vices of government. Public perceptions of health insurance reform reflect a growing sense of skepticism toward the role of government in American society. From 1970 to 2000, the percentage of Americans who trusted "government in Washington to do what is right" only some or none of the time increased from 44 percent to 69 percent. During this period, a majority of Americans also agreed that "government has gone too far in regulating business and interfering with free enterprise."[35] Declining public confidence in government created new challenges for supporters of universal coverage, for each major health insurance reform proposal from the 1970s to the present day sought to increase the role of government in financing health care and regulating the delivery of health care services.

During the 1990s, fears of "big government" emerged as a powerful symbolic enemy for opponents of health care reform. Conservative critics of the Clinton administration's proposed reforms conjured up images of a national health insurance system requiring "such a preposterous Rube Goldberg construction that the great Rube himself wouldn't have had the nerve to put it in the comic strips." In particular, opponents evoked images of an army of government bureaucrats to undermine the legitimacy of universal coverage. Conservatives portrayed the Health Security Act as "a bureaucrat's dream and a patient's nightmare" that would strip physicians of their autonomy and deny patients the right to choose their doctors. Television ads aired by the Health Insurance Association of America (HIAA) warned voters and policy makers that the Clinton administration's "plan forces us to buy our insurance through these new mandatory government health alliances, run by tens of thousands of bureaucrats."[36] Opponents charged that the paternalistic and powerful new bureaucracy required to administer universal coverage would force patients to enroll in a "one size fits all" health plan.

In this narrative, national health insurance marked the end of patient choice and autonomy. Radio commercials sponsored by the HIAA asserted that "Congress is considering legislation that will force us to buy coverage through untested mandatory government health alliances. We may have to give up our current plan for one bought through the Government. Even if we like another plan better, the only ones we can choose are those on the Government list."[37] By mid-1994 opponents of national health insurance successfully redefined the various Democratic reform proposals in the legislative hopper as the first steps down a slippery slope of ever-increasing government regulation.

As a seasoned veteran of policy making in Washington, Senator Robert Dole (R-KS) professed that he was stymied by the bewildering collection of new government agencies required to administer the Clinton Health Security Act. Dole painted a grim picture of the Clinton administration's blueprint for health care reform. "We will have a crisis if we take the President's medicine . . . a massive overdose of government control. . . . Senator Arlen Specter

. . . has prepared a chart of what the health care bureaucracy would look like under the President's plan, and I'd like to show you this chart. It's a great, big chart. It contains 207 boxes. It would take a long time to fully explain it, and frankly, I have difficulty understanding it myself." Dole's colleague Senator Phil Gramm (R-TX)—another leading critic of the administration's reform proposals—echoed this fear of "big government." For Gramm, the fundamental issue in the debate over national health insurance was a simple one: "Americans do not want the Clinton Administration or anybody else telling them what kind of insurance policy they've got to have."[38]

Challenges to the legitimacy of government-led health care reforms resurfaced again over the past decade. During the 2004 presidential campaign, President George W. Bush charged that "the cornerstone" of John Kerry's plan for universal coverage was "to expand the federal government." Bush reaffirmed that "every American has access to high quality, affordable health care," but cautioned voters against "forcing Americans into an expensive, inflexible, one-size-fits-all, government-run health system."[39]

Warnings that a government-run health insurance system will place legions of government bureaucrats between patients and providers also structured opposition to universal coverage in recent years. These same battle-tested narratives about the dangers of big government featured prominently in the 2008 presidential campaign. In particular, opponents of the law targeted government interference in the marketplace for health insurance. During the Republican primaries, Governor Mitt Romney (R-MA) attacked Senator Hillary Clinton's "distrust of markets . . . her distaste for profit-motivated private enterprise . . . and her consequent faith that Washington knows best. The truth is the American people know best, and when a sector of the economy is not working as well as it might, you should look to give the people more influence, to unleash competitive forces, and to welcome private ingenuity. The last thing you should do is apply more government." Romney tapped into long-standing fears about the proper role of government in the health care system and the larger economy. Contrasting Clinton's prescription for more government with his own procompetitive approach, Romney defined his proposal as "the free market way, the private sector way, the individual responsibility way—the American way." As the *Wall Street Journal* editorialized, "Whatever the minor policy differences among Democrats, their major domestic ambition this campaign season is the government takeover of the health care market."[40]

On the campaign trail in 2008, Senator John McCain attacked proposals for a government-run health insurance system. McCain rejected mandated benefits because "that's what big government is all about." The side effects of a "nationalized health care system," McCain warned, would include tax increases, new mandates, and government regulation—in short, "a government monopoly." His opposition to individual and employer mandates underscored the importance of choice as a defining value in health care reform. As McCain declared, "The 'solution' . . . isn't a one size fits all big government takeover of health care. . . . Any 'solution' that robs us of that essential sense of ourselves is a cure far worse than the affliction it is meant to treat."[41]

By urging voters to "preserve the most essential value of American lives— freedom," McCain celebrated the virtues of private solutions to public problems: "We believe that free people may voluntarily unite, but cannot be compelled to do so, and that the limited government that results best protects our individual freedom. In health care, we believe in enhancing the freedom of individuals to receive necessary and desired care. We do not believe in coercion and the use of state power to mandate care, coverage, or costs."[42]

Opposition to national health insurance also energized Republican candidates for Congress in the 2010 midterm elections. Republican candidates adopted a "Pledge to America" that promised swift action to repeal "ObamaCare," arguing that "the new health care law kills jobs, raises taxes, and increases the cost of health care." George Pataki, former governor of New York, declared, "The American people don't want government-run health care and are against ObamaCare for good reason." Pataki's group —Revere America—targeted supporters of the new law in the midterm congressional elections. The group's commercials, run in selected districts, informed voters that "your congressman voted for ObamaCare. Government-run health care. It's a bad plan. Government bureaucrats will benefit. Seniors will get hurt. Costs will go up. Care will go down. Longer waits in doctors' offices. And your right to pick your own physician taken away. It's a plan we didn't want and don't need, but he voted for it anyway. Defeat your congressman."[43]

The complexity of proposals for universal coverage was cited as evidence that such plans were thinly veiled efforts to increase the size and scope of government. House minority leader John Boehner charged that "administration and Congressional Democrats are literally bullying health care groups into cutting backroom deals to fund a government takeover of health care." Senator Mike Enzi (R-WY) echoed these sentiments, arguing that "we need reform, but a government takeover would drive up costs and make the situation worse." That will increase costs and force millions of Americans out of the health care they already have." Conservative critics mobilized opposition to what the *Wall Street Journal* labeled "the worst bill ever" by making its policy tools—from the much-maligned "public option" to state-operated health insurance exchanges—symbols of an overreaching federal government.[44]

Symbolic attacks on national health insurance were particularly effective because they linked opposition to various reform proposals to widely held beliefs in higher-order political symbols such as choice and liberty.[45] By stressing the virtues of private solutions to public problems, opponents of universal coverage also tapped into an underlying cultural shift in recent decades, in which market solutions replaced government regulation as a preferred policy instrument. The continued political appeal of self-reliance—a contemporary version of "rugged individualism"—presented a fundamental challenge for advocates of universal coverage.

Continued skepticism of government constitutes an ongoing threat to the new social compact contained in the PPACA. Cheering the decision of a federal judge in Virginia to toss the mandate, former governor George Allen described the mandate to purchase health insurance as an "unfair, harmful, unconstitutional takeover of health care" and warned that "if the federal government has the power to tell you that you must buy health insurance, then the federal government has the power to force Americans to purchase anything it determines is 'good for you.' Such a government would be unrestrained and omnipotent, and 'we the people' would be less free."[46] Without broad-based, bipartisan agreement on the importance of universal coverage, and the need for government-led initiatives to expand access to health insurance, recent policy changes may be short-lived.

Health insurers and providers warned that a government-run health care system would create unacceptable "side effects" for all Americans each time proposals for universal coverage appeared on the policy agenda. During the 1968 presidential campaign, for example, Richard Nixon opposed a compulsory system of health insurance as a threat to the quality of medical care. Opponents' policy narratives often raised the specter of rationing to undermine support for universal coverage. By bringing millions of new patients into the health care system, critics warned that national health insurance would stretch the existing network of doctors and hospitals beyond capacity, eroding the quality of care for all patients—insured and uninsured alike.[47]

In particular, critics of national health insurance portrayed universal coverage as a threat to patient choice. In this narrative, the price of universal coverage was simply too high. As Senator Robert Dole argued in 1994, "The President's idea is to put a mountain of bureaucrats between you and your doctor. For example, if you are a family member and want to receive care from a specialist or a clinic outside your own state—let's say you live in Kansas and you want to go to Minnesota—then you probably can't do it without asking for approval. And under his plan, information about your health and your treatment can be sent to a national databank without your approval. And that's a compromise of privacy none of us should accept." For their part, physicians claimed that as government sought to control costs by standardizing procedures, regulations and red tape would replace sound medical judgment. In 1994 cardiologists took out a full-page ad in the *New York Times* to remind patients that "nothing is more important than your right to choose your own doctor. Direct, unrestricted access to the heart specialist of your choice could save your life. The debate about health system reform is healthy as long as it doesn't take away your access to the right doctor at the right time."[48]

Elizabeth McCaughey's widely cited article in the *New Republic* argued that passage of the Health Security Act would lead to government control over the practice of medicine. Although the accuracy of her claims was challenged, her dire warnings stuck and were widely reported in the months that followed. Writing in 1994, McCaughey argued, "If the bill passes, you will have to settle for one of the low budget health plans selected by the government. The law will prevent you from going outside the system to buy basic health coverage you think is better, even after you pay the mandatory premium. The bill guarantees you a package of medical services, but you can't have them unless they are deemed 'necessary' and 'appropriate.' That decision will be made by government, not by you and your doctor."[49] Universal coverage, in short, represented the end of patient choice of providers. Doctors and hospitals, for their part, would be hamstrung by a maze of bureaucracy in the wake of reform. The power of McCaughey's attack rested on its use of higher-order symbols such as choice and liberty that were both widely understood and popular with the public. For millions of Americans with private health insurance who were accustomed to choosing their own providers, such warnings raised fears that the quality of their health care would diminish in the wake of reform. Such fears were powerful, for most Americans interact with the health care system on a regular basis; in this context, a loss of choice is not merely an abstract concept, but rather a threat to long-standing, established relationships with health providers.

Similar fear-based appeals raised the specter of outright rationing in 2009. Conservative opponents asked, "Should we risk destroying a system that works for the vast majority to help 15% of the population?" Groups such as Conservatives for Patients' Rights mounted media campaigns to warn Americans that health care reform would create a system where "bureaucrats decide the treatments you receive, the drugs you take, even the doctors you see." Opponents of Democratic proposals for health care reform charged that the law would create "death panels" that would decide which patients would live and which would die. Underlying the rhetoric was the symbolic power of choice and the powerful imagery of personal control over one's own health care. As Representative Eric Cantor (R-VA) argued, "American citizens want to maintain their ability to choose their doctor. They don't want government rationing."[50]

McCaughey reprised her previous attack on the Clinton plan with another scathing critique of Democratic reform proposals in 2009. She argued that within the more than two thousand jargon-laden pages of the bill lurked sinister, little-understood threats to the American health insurance system. While all Americans would be required to enroll in a "qualified plan," McCaughey warned that the definition of what constituted a qualified plan would not be known until more than a year after the passage of the PPACA, "when the secretary of Health and Human Services will decide what a 'qualified plan' covers and how much you'll legally be required to pay for it. That's like a banker telling you to sign the loan agreement now, then filling in the interest rate and repayment terms 18 months later." In addition, McCaughey warned the bill would lead to massive reductions in Medicare funding and new restrictions for patients and providers. "In addition to reducing future Medicare funding by an estimated $500 billion, the bill fundamentally changes how Medicare pays doctors and hospitals, permitting the government to dictate treatment decisions."[51]

For the past four decades, opponents of national health insurance also characterized universal coverage as an expensive boondoggle. In the early 1970s, the Nixon administration argued the cost of Senator Edward Kennedy's proposed Health Security Act was "equal to about half the total present general revenues of the Federal Government and would be equivalent to a Federal health tax of over $1,000 a year for every household in the United

States." The threat of tax increases was a potent symbol for opponents of reform and appealed to deep-seated American concerns about the cost of government. The 1972 Republican Party platform reaffirmed opposition to "nationalized compulsory health insurance" on the grounds that it "would at least triple in taxes the amount the average citizen now pays for health."[52] In a society with a long-standing suspicion of taxation, such charges were designed to raise important doubts about the ability to pay for reform.

The deficit-driven policy-making environment of the early 1990s ensured that the projected cost of comprehensive health care reform featured prominently in policy debates. As the chair of the Republican National Committee charged in 1994, "We can't afford a government-run health care system financed by a massive payroll tax." Opponents defined universal coverage as a drain on the economy and a millstone around the neck of American businesses. In this story of decline, government-mandated health insurance would lower the rate of economic growth and increase unemployment. As the National Federation of Independent Business framed the issue, "What's more important—the job or the health insurance?"[53]

Once again, critics of health insurance reform turned to familiar stories of decline to challenge the affordability of universal coverage in 2009. Representative Paul Ryan (R-WI) charged that Democratic proposals for reform were "the absolute height of fiscal irresponsibility. . . . The shame of it all is that we could actually fix what's broken in health care without breaking what's working, and without creating a huge new entitlement program that will accelerate the bankruptcy of this country." Conservatives charged that in its effort to enact health care reform, Congress was rushing toward "fiscal suicide" and accused supporters of reform of "using every budget gimmick and trick in the book: Leave out inconvenient spending, back load spending to disguise the true scale . . . promise spending cuts to doctors and hospitals that have no record of materializing, and so on." Senator Mike Enzi railed against reform, charging that "for millions of Americans, the government run plan would turn into a bureaucratic nightmare, with the efficiency and customer service of the Department of Motor Vehicles or the IRS. Washington bureaucrats would literally decide whether patients would live or die by rationing newer, more expensive therapies."[54]

Business groups purchased full-page advertisements in newspapers to oppose "expensive new mandates [that] will result in lost jobs, lower wages, less flexibility, and higher health care costs. . . . [T]he bill imposes a staggering $527 billion in new taxes. These taxes will devastate many small businesses—the engine of job creation in America. . . . This fatally flawed and irresponsible bill should be taken back to the drawing board immediately. It's a bill American businesses and working families can't afford to pay." Reformers had hoped that reform would be a feather in their cap, but the reality was far different. Less than six months after its passage, opponents pilloried the new law. "Higher health care costs. Cuts to seniors' health care. Higher taxes, penalties, and fines on employers that keep them from creating the new jobs we need. These are the realities of ObamaCare."[55] In a remarkable twist, many Democratic candidates for Congress touted their votes against health care reform on the eve of the midterm elections.

The Road Ahead

For the majority of the public, dire warnings of a health care crisis are at odds with their own personal experiences with the health care system. The stories of crisis told by reformers are an unwitting impediment to reform. When the predicted collapse or meltdown of the health insurance fails to materialize, reformers' cries of crisis seem hollow. In this context, calls for a significantly expanded role for government to address the crisis appear either unnecessary or counterproductive for insured Americans.

As a rhetorical strategy, the imagery of crisis fell short on several counts. Americans are undeniably concerned about the financial and personal costs of illness, but narratives of crisis fail to acknowledge that the power of this message varies according to individual circumstances. Although access to care was a growing problem for millions of Americans over the past four decades, the ranks of the uninsured increased steadily—year after year— without a clear "tipping point." The growing number of uninsured was a symptom of a long-term, systemic change in the way Americans obtained health insurance; as the employer-based health insurance system began to fray in recent years, millions of working families no longer had access to affordable coverage. Crisis rhetoric, however, fails to capture this long-term secular trend. In particular, the symbolic potency of the struggles facing uninsured families was less immediate for the 85 percent of Americans who are covered by health insurance. Access to care was an acute problem for the uninsured, but three out of four Americans—regardless of sex, race, or income—remained satisfied with the quality of their care. If Beatrix Hoffman is correct that "health care activism is rooted in people's experiences with the health care system," this underlying satisfaction with health insurers and health providers presents a substantial obstacle for reformers.[56]

For much of the twentieth century, campaigns for national health insurance and Medicare captured the imagination of the public by tapping into deeply held beliefs in fairness, equality, and progress. These narratives used progress as an organizing principle for health care reform and promised reforms that built upon the strengths of the existing system rather than seeking to replace it. Daily coverage of medical discoveries, new treatments, and a growing body of evidence that Americans were living longer, healthier lives lent credibility to this policy narrative. Such stories struck a responsive chord with the public—particularly the insured public—far more than the wide-eyed warnings of crisis offered by supporters of universal coverage.

Most crisis narratives, in contrast, were not anchored by higher-order political symbols such as freedom, equality, or efficiency. Instead, reformers sought to demonstrate the scope and severity of the emerging crisis through the recitation of endless statistics, horror stories, and dire predictions of future trends. In 2009–10, for example, Democrats became bogged down in a complex, mind-numbing debate about the nuances of policy, arguing over the details of health insurance exchanges, the "public option," and other situational symbols. When these stories clashed with Americans' lived experiences with the health insurance system—as they inevitably did—crisis talk lost traction with the public.

As a description of what ails the American health care system, crisis narratives fail to capture the daily interactions of most Americans with doctors, insurers, and other caregivers. Surveying five decades of public opinion polls on health care reform, Robert Blendon concluded that while "most of the public has never been completely satisfied with the system, . . . never has a majority supported developing an alternative system." Despite extensive attention to health care reform during the 2008 presidential campaign, fewer than one in five Americans agreed that the US health care system was "in a state of crisis." Since most Americans did not believe that the health insurance system was in danger of an imminent collapse, calls for reform failed to resonate strongly with insured Americans. Although a majority of the public believed the system had "major problems," such an assessment lacked the symbolic power contained in warnings of an imminent crisis. From 1982 to 2002, the notion that "the health care system has so much wrong with it that we need to completely rebuild it" was never endorsed by most Americans.[57]

More generally, as a concept, crisis became commonplace, thereby undermining its symbolic power. As George Will notes, "Our government declares war promiscuously—on cancer, drugs, environmental problems, etc.—but never when actually going to war."[58] In a similar vein, reformers have taken to describing every social problem as a crisis. The overuse of *crisis* to describe events of varying severity cheapens and devalues its ability to mobilize the public; if everything can be framed as a crisis, the urgency associated with the term is lost.

Instead, continued cries of crisis inadvertently opened the door for a counternarrative by opponents of reform that questioned the very existence of a health insurance crisis in America. Descriptions of a "crumbling" or "collapsing" health care system raised public anxieties, but in the absence of a "meltdown," critics argued that the desperate stories of uninsured patients were overblown and did not represent the experience of most Americans. By the early 1970s, more than 90 percent of population under the age of sixty-five had some form of private health insurance coverage, leading many observers to conclude that the steady growth of Blue Cross made national health insurance unnecessary. Businesses, health insurers, and health providers accentuated the positive features of the American health insurance system, while downplaying its shortcomings. In 1974, for example, the president of the American Medical Association described the state of the US health system as fundamentally sound and declared that the "health crisis" had been "trumped up" by politicians. Insurance industry officials employed a similar strategy, conceding that "repairs to the system are needed, but nothing that would justify total federal funding or a federal bureaucracy to run all health matters in America."[59] The present system, in short, worked well for most Americans.

Similar arguments resurfaced during the heated debate over the Clinton administration's Health Security Act. In 1994—after two years of extensive congressional debate over health care reform—many Republicans continued to dispute reformers' claims that the health insurance system faced a crisis. As Senate minority leader Robert Dole argued in an interview with CNN in December 1993, "Too many of us in politics are trying to make a crisis out of something that's not a crisis. . . . And I think there's a feeling out there that there's been this intense—every day, every day—push to get people to accept the feeling that there's a crisis in America in health care."[60]

Senator Dole emerged as the leading proponent of this "no crisis" view during the debate over the Clinton administration's proposed Health Security Act. In his televised response to President Clinton's State of the Union address in 1994, Dole declared, "America has the best health care system in the world. . . . [P]eople from every corner of the globe come here when they need the very best treatment, and . . . our goal should be to insure that every American has access to this system. . . . Our country has health care problems, but not a health care crisis." Dole forcefully reiterated this message as the Senate began its debate over health care reform in 1994: "America has the best health care system in the world. America has the best health care delivery system in the world. America has the best health care delivery system in the world. And I repeat it three times because I'm concerned that actions we might take in this chamber in the next couple of weeks or so will mean those words are no longer true." Personalizing the issue for his colleagues, Dole argued that "a lot of people have experienced miracles in health care in America, and I've been fortunate to be one of those. And had I returned home from World War II to any other nation, I'm not certain what would have happened to me."[61] Dole's rebuttal was anchored in a belief in American exceptionalism. By celebrating the virtues of the American health insurance system, yet acknowledging the need for incremental reform, critics offered a reassuring alternative to the rhetoric of crisis that reflected Americans' belief in the possibilities of progress.

Supporters of universal coverage must learn an important lesson from decades of opposition to national health insurance. Reformers need a better policy story. As David Blumenthal observed more than a decade ago, proponents of reform must persuade Americans to "overcome their innate skepticism of government and agree to entrust it with new authority over the financing of a vital, personal service." Despite decades of crisis talk, no grassroots social movement has taken root to demand universal coverage. Debates over health insurance reform are defined by a fundamental question: what role should government play in organizing, and financing, health care in America? Reformers ignore this question at their peril, for each debate over health care reform—from World War I to the present day—ultimately turned on this question. In the early to mid-twentieth century, concerns about government's role were framed in terms of socialism, as opponents contrasted the virtues of private, voluntary solutions—the "American way"—with unfamiliar, "socialistic" compulsory schemes. As the fear of socialism waned in the late twentieth century, "big government" replaced concerns about socialism as an organizing principle, but the underlying policy question about the role of government remained. Debates over the health insurance reform in the early 1990s, and again in 2009–10, failed to confront this fundamental proposition. In the end, this is the most egregious example of the "unintended misuse" of language, for by framing public discussion of health insurance reform using the rhetoric of crisis, reformers missed the opportunity to connect universal coverage to core American values such as equal treatment, fairness, justice, and positive notions of liberty.[62]

Forging a consensus over values must precede efforts to lobby for specific policy proposals. Too often, reformers have skipped this step and moved directly to consideration of the specific merits of competing reform plans. Advocates of universal coverage must move beyond the rhetoric of crisis and must instead anchor calls for expanded access to health care in widely held social beliefs. Such a conversation is a necessary condition for establishing a long-term, stable system of universal coverage, for providing coverage to all Americans cannot be accomplished without affecting the status quo for insured individuals. As James Mongan and Thomas Lee note, "If broad access to health care is ever to be more than a campaign sound bite, it cannot be a casual commitment. Americans must understand that they are going to make real sacrifices for other Americans." The challenge for reformers today remains the same as it was in 1971, when Senator Jacob Javits (D-NY) declared that policy makers needed to "arouse the conscience of the Nation to join together in a common effort to . . . develop a better and universal system of health care for every American."[63]

A Second Opinion

The danger [communism] poses promises to be of an indefinite duration. To meet it successfully, there is called for, not so much the emotional and transitory sacrifices of crisis, but rather those which enable us to carry forward steadily, surely and without complaint the burdens of a prolonged and complex struggle.　　　　　　　　　　　　　　　　—Dwight D. Eisenhower,
"Farewell Address to the American People," 1961

THE CHALLENGES FACING the American health care system today are similar to the national security threats described by Dwight Eisenhower in his farewell address to the American people. The American health care system resembles a patient suffering from multiple degenerative conditions (for example, hypertension, high cholesterol, acid reflux, and osteoarthritis) that must be treated in a coordinated fashion. As Lawrence Brown observes, although the American health care system is "deeply dysfunctional by most standards," it "remains disturbingly stable."[1] Few providers, payers, or patients are fully satisfied with the status quo, but the problems described in the preceding chapters are chronic, not acute, conditions. The challenge for policy makers lies not in finding a cure for rising costs, uneven quality, and unequal access to health care, but rather in managing and controlling these chronic conditions.

The cries of crisis that framed public deliberation over health care reform since the late 1960s contributed to a dysfunctional discourse. *Crisis,* as it is used to frame health care debates, is an example of what George Orwell termed a "meaningless word" that lacks precision. Neither those who use the concept nor their intended audience agrees upon the real meaning of the crisis. This problem is hardly confined to health care, for as Orwell noted in the case of democracy, "not only is there no agreed definition, but the attempt to make one is resisted from all sides." Policy debates revolve around the construction of meanings. Issue entrepreneurs, interest groups, and public officials seek to explain the scope, significance, and root causes of policy problems to build support for their preferred solutions. To do so, they often turn to metaphor. Metaphors, however, can clarify or confuse. Writing of the response to the 9/11 terrorist attacks, Hendrick Hertzberg observed that "the metaphor of war . . . ascribes to the perpetrators a dignity that they do not merit, a status they cannot claim, and a strength they do not possess. Worse, it points toward a set of responses that could prove futile or counterproductive."[2] In a similar fashion, crisis talk misconstrues the nature of the policy challenges facing reformers, who must build support for long-term management of the chronic problems plaguing the American health care system.

Crisis narratives continued to frame public deliberation about health care reform in 2012. In its brief submitted to the US Supreme Court in advance of the *Department of Health and Human Services v. State of Florida,* the Obama administration defended the Patient Protection and Affordable Care Act on the grounds that it was enacted "to address a crisis in the national health care market."[3] Repeated cries of crisis, however, suffer from a credibility gap. The underlying stability of the system, despite its problems, diminishes the potency of crisis as a call to action, for the dire depictions of a collapsing system fail to mesh with the daily reality experienced by most Americans. Each day, most Americans who need to use the health care system do so without incident. Despite decades of crisis talk, no identifiable "tipping point" exists to compel policy makers to take action. Instead, the chronic problems of rising costs, preventable medical errors and patient deaths, and uneven access to care worsen slowly, often imperceptibly over time. Despite the system's shortcomings, many of these ailments are not immediately apparent to most Americans who use the health care system.

As a result, cries of crisis remain unpersuasive. Nearly two years after the passage of the Affordable Care Act, more Americans viewed the law unfavorably than favorably, and only one in four Americans believed that they would be "better off" after the implementation of health care reform. Rather than providing a catalyst for change, crisis narratives contain the seeds of their undoing. When the predicted "meltdown" fails to materialize, the rationale for reform becomes suspect. As Eli Ginzberg noted in 1990, "Steadily rising health care costs are burdensome and sooner or later will become intolerable," but "no one can be certain of the point of no return." Although crisis talk promises short-term political advantages, the irony of crisis talk is that repeated warnings of imminent collapse actually become a roadblock for reformers. Without a clearly identifiable point of no return, it is difficult to keep loosely knit reform coalitions together. Warnings that the rate of health care spending, the number of uninsured Americans, or the shortage of nurses is "unsustainable" lack traction with policy makers and the public, for as Jon

Oberlander observes, "We cannot know in advance what the breaking point is, or if we are going to get there."[4]

Crisis narratives also fail to capture the daily experiences of most Americans with the health care system. Perceptions of the health care system reflect individual experiences. All Americans are not affected equally by rising health care costs, malpractice, or the availability of health insurance. Insured patients, for example, often view talk of a crisis of access as someone else's problem. Similarly, warnings of a medical malpractice crisis have more traction in certain high-risk states than elsewhere. Despite decades of dire warnings that the health care system was on the brink of collapse, most Americans remain highly satisfied with their interactions with health care providers. In 2008, for example, eight in ten Americans rated the medical care they received as "good" or "excellent." Furthermore, fewer than one in five Americans described the health care system as "in crisis," compared to nearly half (45 percent) who believed that the United States had the "best health care system" in the world.[5] Such high levels of satisfaction with health care services are inconsistent with the notion that the US health care system is on the brink of collapse.

The most significant shortcoming of crisis rhetoric, however, is that it is ill-suited to mobilize public support for what Eisenhower described as a "prolonged and complex struggle." No quick fixes exist for long-term, chronic problems such as rising costs, medical errors, the shortage of health providers, and the uninsured. To tackle our most pressing problems, supporters of reform must first focus public attention on the need for change and then persuade the public that change is both possible and desirable. If fear-based narratives of crisis fail to resonate with voters, the proper prescription for reformers is a new rhetorical strategy that builds upon widely shared values and beliefs in American political culture.

A Question of Governability

Events in recent years persuaded many observers that the American political process is broken. Health care reform became an exemplar of what's wrong with American policy making. As *USA Today* editorialized in 2009, "In health care politics, down is up, right is left, and the sun rises each morning in the West." Public deliberation about the Patient Protection and Affordable Care Act, for example, raised fundamental questions about the nation's ability to address difficult social problems. After months of acerbic debate in Congress over health care reform, President Barack Obama defined the success of health care reform as a key test of policy makers' ability to govern the nation. "At stake right now," the president declared, "is not just our ability to solve this problem, but our ability to solve any problem." The passage of reform in March 2010 did little to assuage the concerns of critics about the policy-making capacity of American political institutions. After the final vote on health care reform in 2010 failed to garner support from any Republican legislators, many observers wondered aloud whether compromise on difficult policy issues was still possible. In an era of divided government dominated by growing polarization and decreased bipartisanship, critics wondered whether it was possible to govern effectively.[6]

Doubts about the problem-solving capacity of American political institutions are now widespread. In recent years, news reports compared Congress to a "fight club" where compromise was seen as a sign of capitulation. Long-standing members of Congress bemoaned that "we are becoming more coarse and divided here."[7] Such concerns, of course, are not new. Compromise is difficult in the context of a Congress characterized by growing ideological polarization. On the Right, the rise of the Tea Party movement in 2010 fed off popular discontent with, and distrust of, government, while the Occupy Wall Street protests (which spread around the nation in 2011) signified growing dissatisfaction with the political process among the Left. Declining faith in the policy-making institutions, and in political leaders, is evident in public opinion polls and news coverage.

Although American politics is increasingly polarized, the nature, extent, and consequences of this polarization remain in dispute. Morris Fiorina, for example, contends that both decision makers and interest groups have become increasingly disconnected from the values and beliefs of average Americans since the 1970s. While the public remains moderate, and largely disengaged from partisan bickering within the Beltway, sharp—and growing—partisan and ideological divisions among the "political class" preclude compromise on most issues. Others, however, argue that cultural, geographic, ideological, and partisan differences have widened significantly within the mass public since the 1970s. The result, argue many observers, is an increasingly dysfunctional political process incapable of discussing issues in a civil manner, let alone brokering compromises.[8] Whether the disjunction occurs between voters and their elected representatives, or within the public itself, reformers must identify ways to find common ground to address the chronic problems plaguing the American health care system.

Recent complaints about the inability of political institutions to tackle difficult policy challenges bear an uncanny resemblance to dire warnings issued by policy makers and pundits four decades ago. In the 1970s, academic observers questioned the ability of governments to successfully manage economic, fiscal, and urban problems. Talk of a "governability crisis" raised fundamental questions about the problem-solving capacity of American political institutions. As Samuel Huntington observes, "In the United States, as elsewhere in the industrialized world, domestic problems thus become intractable problems. The public develops expectations which it is impossible for government to meet. The activities—and expenditures—of government expand, but the success of government in achieving its goals seems dubious." The roots of the crisis, Huntington argues, could be found in two contradictory trends: "a substantial increase in governmental activity and a substantial decrease in governmental authority." After President Jimmy Carter declared that America was plagued by a "national malaise" in a nationally televised address in 1979, many observers worried that the nation faced a crisis of confidence. "The fundamental question," as James Sundquist wrote, was "whether in the next few years the U.S. government can be made to work—under any leadership. The crisis of confidence turns out to be a crisis of efficacy, or competence, in government. After the shocks the country has suffered, can a series of successes follow?"[9] Events in 2011 renewed questions about whether elected officials and institutions could still govern. In the wake of stalemates over deficit reduction and the collapse of the "super-committee" in the fall of 2011, partisan brinkmanship on raising the debt ceiling, and a continued impasse over entitlement reform, the critiques of both the news media and political pundits bore an uncanny resemblance to earlier discussions of a governability crisis in the 1970s.

Health care reformers today have much to learn from earlier eras. The roots of both ongoing policy stalemates and continued challenges to the need for comprehensive health care reform are linked to the rhetoric of reform. Reformers must restore faith in the ability of government to solve social problems. As Gerald Seib noted in 2009, the health care debate "is so intense because it's not really about health care at all. On a deeper level it's about the role of government in America's economy."[10] Too often, reformers failed to recognize this basic fact and dismissed charges that health care reform would lead to a new era of "big government" or "socialism" as mere hyperbole. They are not. Health care reform raises fundamental questions about the role government should play, not just in financing health care, but also in regulating relationships among patients, providers, and health insurers.

A New Prescription for Health Care Reform

The politics of fear has fractured and frustrated reform for decades. The political appeal of fear in public discourse is understandable, for health care brings together several of the most potent and enduring sources of fear, including fears of death, disability, and suffering. Fear, as John Hollander notes, is "the fundamental emotion, driving other drives."[11] Proposals to reform the health care system often arouse fears of change (for example, diminished choice or limits on personal liberty). The presence of nagging, chronic fears in health policy debates often focuses public attention on worst-case scenarios and horror stories in an effort to dramatize the need for swift and decisive action. The use of fear, however, comes with a high cost. Even when fears of a collapsing health care system prove to be unfounded, their corrosive effects remain, sowing seeds of doubt among those who use the health care system and who depend on it to earn a living.

To address the chronic problems facing the American health care system, reformers must move beyond narratives of crisis to tell a new policy story. As Walter Fisher observes, "Any political rhetoric will remain viable as long as historical circumstances permit, as long as there is not an equally compelling story and character to confront it and to show its ultimate lack of coherence and fidelity."[12] The circumstances are ripe to remove the rhetorical roadblocks that continue to stymie efforts to build support for long-term, sustainable reforms. Reformers must persuade a skeptical public that not only is it possible to make difficult choices, but government has a meaningful role in reshaping the health care system.

One of the most significant roadblocks for health care reform is what James Morone describes as Americans' enduring "dread of government." This dread was evident in recent opposition to health care reform. In 2010 former House Speaker Newt Gingrich warned that "centralized planning inherently leads to dictatorship, which is why having a secular socialist machine try to impose government run health care in this country is such a significant step away from freedom and away from liberty, and towards a government-dominated society." Opposition reflected lingering doubts about the proper role of government in the health care system. "The problem with Obama-Care," Representative Joe Pitts (R-PA) wrote, "is that it is a big government solution to a problem created by big government. . . . ObamaCare is creating

159 new federal offices and tens of thousands of new regulations." The result, Pitts argued, is that "bureaucrats will make decisions that should be left to doctors and patients."[13]

For some, the future of health care reform rests upon a communitarian view of health and health care. Lawrence Wallack and Regina Lawrence, for example, urged reformers to embrace a new "language of interconnectedness" built upon "egalitarian and humanitarian values, of interdependence and community." Communitarians emphasize policies to promote the "common good," in contrast to the partisan pulling and hauling of interest-group politics.[14] Calls to embrace policies that foster the common good—even when bolstered by moral and theological arguments—still face practical challenges to persuade the public to embrace changes in how health care is organized, paid for, and accessed. A new narrative is needed that both exhorts Americans to raise their expectations for health care reform and reassures the public. Health care reformers, in short, must answer a question similar to the one posed by Ronald Reagan to voters in 1980: will you be better off after reform than you are today? If the public answers in the affirmative, reform is possible, if not guaranteed. If voters see health care reform as a threat to their well-being, however, its future is uncertain at best.

Communitarian appeals often lack traction in an intensely individualistic society. Although laudable, the communitarian prescription fails to acknowledge the power of self-interest in American political life. Few Americans will endorse policies that do not promise improvement over the status quo. The passage of the Patient Protection and Affordable Care Act underscored the importance of self-interest in debates over health care reform. This long-awaited triumph of American liberalism contained a hidden irony. On the eve of reform, public opinion polls revealed that a majority of Americans believed the bill would hurt the quality of health care. Soon after its passage, opponents filed suit to block the implementation of the new law in federal court, and dissatisfaction over the reform contributed to a midterm rout for congressional Democrats in 2010. A year after its passage, health care reform illustrated the growing polarization in American politics, as 71 percent of Democrats held a favorable view of the law, compared to only 9 percent of Republicans. Most Americans remained deeply skeptical of, if not openly opposed to, many of its key provisions. Regardless of age, income, or insurance status, fewer than half of all Americans had a favorable opinion of the bill. Remarkably, support for the bill was lower among the uninsured (36 percent) than among Americans with health insurance (43 percent).

After the passage of health care reform, a majority of the public also believed that the quality of health care would either stay the same or get worse.[15] In the end, public opinion polls demonstrate the shortcomings of public deliberation about health care reform, for despite two years of intense debates, the public remains unconvinced of the need for reform.

To craft a more persuasive policy narrative, reformers must return to the stories of progress that defined previous campaigns for health care reform in the twentieth century. The success of health care reform, in the long run, rests on the ability of policy makers to persuade the public that they will be better off in the wake of reform. Narratives of progress appeal to self-interest by offering hope to all Americans that health care reform will improve their own interactions with the health care system. Patients and providers, for example, stand to benefit in concrete ways from efforts to reduce medical errors and enhance patient safety. From well-organized medical subspecialties to trade organizations representing medical device manufacturers and pharmaceutical companies and a wide range of disease advocacy groups, the American health care system is organized around self-interest. Reformers ignore these interests as their own peril. Successful health care reform must address the hopes and fears of average Americans about their own interactions with the health care system. Elements of each narrative appeared during each debate over health care reform from the 1960s to the present day but were subsumed—or shuffled aside—by cries of crisis.

Reframing Costs as Investments

The first narrative defines health care reform as an investment, not a crisis. Progress in health care is a familiar story line and also reflects the enduring appeal of efficiency as an organizing principle for reform. The public is well acquainted with innovations that promise to extend life or improve the quality of life for patients. Stories of new scientific advances, promising treatments, and transformational technologies appeal to the self-interest of patients and providers alike. A safer health care system, for example, offers tangible benefits for all patients. In a similar vein, training additional nurses, and improving their salaries and working conditions, benefits all Americans who use health care services. The notion of health care reform as an investment enjoyed a high level of narrative fidelity with the public, for the rapid pace of medical innovation paid handsome dividends in medical treatments and improved outcomes during the twentieth century.[16]

Previous campaigns for reform also framed health care as an investment in better health. Additional spending on health insurance for the elderly and poor, for hospital construction, and on biomedical research enjoyed widespread bipartisan support in the decades following World War II. Each program offered tangible evidence of the return on the nation's investment in health care in communities across America. Stories of progress build upon this vision of better health care for all Americans by improving access to health insurance, reducing medical errors, and ensuring an adequate supply of nurses to care for the sick. Surveying twenty-five years of public opinion from 1973 to 1998, Robert Blendon notes that fewer than one out of ten Americans believed that the nation was spending "too much" on health care.[17]

Health Care Reform as Social Justice

Americans also profess strong support for the idea of equality in health care. In this narrative, health care reform is a matter of simple justice. Stories of injustice—whether of sick families unable to obtain care, nursing shortages, or the challenges facing patients and families who suffer from medical errors—are essential tools for reformers. Such stories challenge the conscience of society. Stories of unnecessary suffering, or even death, as Atul Gawande observes, become "unconscionable in any society that purports to serve the needs of ordinary people, and at some alchemical point, they combine with opportunity and leadership to produce change." The message for reformers is clear: "Advocates of universal health insurance need to remind not only themselves, but also their fellow citizens, of the moral and ethical roots of their position."[18]

Unlike the rhetoric of crisis, narratives of equality tap into deeply rooted social and political values. As Daniel Yankelovich notes, "The majority of Americans have not become morally obtuse." This theme can be found in recent debates over health care reform. As President Barack Obama declared at the signing of the Children's Health Insurance Program renewal in 2009, "We're not a nation that leaves struggling families to fend for themselves, especially when they've done everything right. . . . In a decent society, there are certain obligations that are not subject to tradeoffs or negotiations, and health care for our children is one of these obligations." This underlying sense of morality within the public creates an opportunity to help Americans "face the real human costs imposed on our fellow citizens by the confusion and neglect inherent in America's high cost health care system."[19] Redefining the imagery of reform from crisis to equality is not simply a lexical shift, but rather a fundamental change in strategy. This narrative enables all patients—rich or poor, insured or uninsured—to reflect upon their personal experiences with care as they reflect upon the type of health care system that is most consistent with American values.

Ironically, the future of health care reform may depend on an important lesson from the Reagan era. Reagan's election—and his subsequent legislative successes during his first term—dispelled the myth that the nation was ungovernable. As a candidate, Reagan campaigned on a clear, concise platform that focused on downsizing government (for example, cutting taxes, raising defense spending, slashing social welfare programs). Less than two years after Carter's malaise speech, Reagan demonstrated—forcefully—that nonincremental policy change was still possible by passing a sweeping set of economic reforms. Both Democrats and Republicans alike continue to evoke Reagan's presidency as a watershed moment in twentieth-century American politics. As Barack Obama declared, "Ronald Reagan changed the trajectory of America in a way that Richard Nixon did not and in a way that Bill Clinton did not. He put us on a fundamentally different path." Change came, not through an electoral realignment, but through a rhetorical one. As Nicholas Lemann argues, "Reagan's critical contribution was to change the terms of the debate."[20]

In the end, the success of health care reform depends upon the ability of policy makers to convince a skeptical public that progress is not only possible but also consistent with American ideals. Reformers must persuade Americans to suspend their doubts, if not outright hostility, toward government. Just as Ronald Reagan reshaped Americans' ideas about the size, and role, of government, reformers must change the terms of debate over health care reform. The only way to deal with chronic, sustained problems facing the American health care system is to forge agreement among a diverse group of stakeholders. Viewed in this light, rhetoric is not incidental but central to reform. A new rhetoric of reform acknowledges the power of self-interest and appeals to the power of hope, not fear, to mobilize public support for health care reform. Ultimately, the "challenge of leadership is to make people believe again that government can make a difference."[21]

NOTES

INTRODUCTION   Constructing the Health Care Crisis

1. Robin Toner, "Poll Says Public Favors Changes in Health Policy," *New York Times,* April 6, 1993, A1; Timothy Johnson, "Town with a Heart: Small Town Fights Health Care Crisis," *20/20,* December 26, 2003.

2. See Bruce Kuklick, *The Good Ruler: From Herbert Hoover to Richard Nixon;* Thomas Langston, *With Reverence and Contempt;* Daniel T. Rodgers, *Contested Truths: Keywords in American Politics Since Independence;* and Rita Charon, "Narrative Medicine: A Model for Empathy, Reflection, Profession, and Trust," 1898.

3. Robert Alford, "The Political Economy of Health Care: Dynamics Without Change"; Godfrey Hodgson, "The Politics of America Health Care: What Is It Costing You?"; Stephen Shortell and Walter McNerney, "Criteria and Guidelines for Reforming the U.S. Health Care System."

4. Cindy Jajich-Toth and Burns W. Roper, "Americans' Views on Health Care: A Study in Contradictions"; Robert J. Blendon et al., "Americans' Health Priorities: Curing Cancer and Controlling Costs"; Jon Gabel, Howard Cohen, and Steven Fink, "Americans' Views on Health Care: Foolish Inconsistencies?"; ABC News/Kaiser Family Foundation/USA Today, *Health Care in America 2006 Survey Chartpack;* Robert J. Blendon and John Benson, "Understanding How Americans View Health Care Reform"; Everett Carl Ladd, "The Congress Problem"; Lawrence Brown, "Comparing Health Systems in Four Countries: Lessons for the United States," 55.

5. Joel Best, *Random Violence: How We Talk About New Crimes and New Victims.*

6. James A. Morone, "Nativism, Hollow Corporations, and Managed Competition: Why the Clinton Health Care Reform Failed," 391.

7. P. M. S. Hacker, *Wittgenstein,* 9.

8. "The Real Health Issue," *New York Times,* June 25, 1974, 36; Linda Disch, "Publicity-Stunt Participation and Sound Bite Polemics: The Health Care Debate, 1993–94," 7; Daniel Yankelovich, "The Debate That Wasn't: The Public and the Clinton Health Care Plan"; William Glaberson, "Struggling to Bring the Health-Care Debate Home to Readers," *New York Times,* May 25, 1993, A2; Theodore R. Marmor, "A Summer of Discontent: Press Coverage of Murder and Medical Care Reform," 499.

9. Kathy Kiely and John Fritze, "Passions Flare Up at Health Care Forums," *USA Today,* August 10, 2009, A4; Bob Beckel and Cal Thomas, "How to Break Up Town Brawls," *USA Today,* August 20, 2009, A11; Bill Lambrecht, "Tempers Run High at Forums on Reform of Health Care," *Providence Sunday Journal,* August 9, 2009, C12; Nancy Pelosi and Steny Hoyer, "'Un-American' Attacks Can't Derail Health Care Debate," *USA Today,* August 10, 2009, A7; "Dishonest Debate Mars Bid to Overhaul Health Care," *USA Today,* July 31, 2009, A10.

10. Murray Edelman, *The Symbolic Uses of Politics.*

11. Charon, "Narrative Medicine," 1897.

12. Beatrix Hoffman, *The Wages of Sickness;* Robert B. Hackey, "Symbolic Politics and Health Care Reform in the 1940s and 1990s"; "Text of President's Message to Congress Advocating Passage of Medical Care Bill," *New York Times,* February 28, 1962, 16.

13. Richard M. Nixon, "Remarks at a Briefing on the Nation's Health System."

14. Hodgson, "Politics of America Health Care"; William L. Kissick, "Health Policy Directions for the 1970s," 1343; David Kotelchuck, "The Health Status of Americans," 5.

15. Kuklick, *Good Ruler,* 30.

16. John Edwards, "Press Release: Edwards Announces Plan for Universal Health Care"; John McCain, "Text of McCain Speech on Health Care," *Wall Street Journal,* October 11, 2007.

17. Harold M. Schmeck, "A Plan to Insure Health Care for All," *New York Times,* July 12, 1970, E5; Harry Smith and Lester Holt, "The Health Care Crisis in Chicago," *CBS This Morning,* July 10, 1990. See also David C. Colby and Timothy Cook, "Epidemics and Agendas: The Politics of Nightly News Coverage of AIDS."

18. John M. Broder, Robert Pear, and Milt Freudenheim, "Problem of Lost Health Benefits Is Reaching into the Middle Class," *New York Times,* November 25, 2002, A1; "The No. 1 Worry," *Des Moines Register,* October 12, 2004; "Health Care Reform: A Pill Too Bitter for U.S. to Swallow," *USA Today,* October 17, 2006, 17.

19. Joseph Turow and Rachel Gans, *As Seen on TV: Health Policy Issues in TV's Medical Dramas;* Allison Waldman, "Dramas Deliver Medical Messages: Fiction Programming Can Create Awareness of Health Care, Diseases"; Victoria Rideout, *Television as a Health Educator: A Case Study of "Grey's Anatomy";* Candace Cummins Gauthier, "Television Drama and Popular Film as Medical Narrative"; Mollyann Brodie et al., "Communicating Health Information Through the Entertainment Media."

20. David Denby, "Calculating Rhythm," 90.

21. This episode first aired during season 2 of *Extreme Makeover: Home Edition* (episode 20, "The Harvey Family") on April 24, 2005. For an episode summary, see http://abc.go.com/shows/extreme-makeover-home-edition/episode-detail/harvey-family/68111 (accessed December 23, 2011).

22. Deborah Stone and Theodore Marmor, "Introduction," 255; Shortell and McNerney, "Criteria and Guidelines," 463.

23. Patricia Roberts-Miller, "Democracy, Demagoguery, and Critical Rhetoric," 459; Lawrence R. Jacobs, "Health Reform Impasse: The Politics of American Ambivalence Toward Government," 643.

ONE   The Rhetoric of Health Care Reform

1. Virginia Woolf, "Mr. Bennett and Mrs. Brown."

2. "50% More Doctors Urged by Parran," *New York Times,* October 10, 1947, 29.

3. "Text of President's Message to Congress Advocating Passage of Medical Care Bill," *New York Times,* February 28, 1962, 16.

4. Godfrey Hodgson, *America in Our Time,* 6, 464.

5. "60,995,000 Listed in Hospital Plans," *New York Times,* August 18, 1949, 23; "50% More Doctors Urged by Parran"; "121,000,000 in U.S. Now Carry Insurance Against Cost of Hospital and Doctor Bills," *New York Times,* January 12, 1959, 93.

6. "Johnson's Special Message to Congress Outlining Broad National Health Program," *New York Times,* January 8, 1965, 16.

7. Quoted in Kuklick, *Good Ruler,* 139.

8. Donald Light, "Sociological Perspectives on Competition in Health Care," 969.

9. Hodgson, *America in Our Time,* 3; Rick Perlstein, *Nixonland;* Hodgson, *America in Our Time,* 15 (emphasis in the original).

10. Albert O. Hirschman, *Shifting Involvements,* 40.

11. Burton Klein, "The Limits to Growth: A Report for the Club of Rome."

12. Robert P. Hart et al., *Political Keywords: Using Language That Uses Us,* 5; Murray Edelman, *Constructing the Political Spectacle,* 31; Ronald Rotunda, *The Politics of Language,* 9. In *Nixonland,* Perlstein uses Nixon's ascendance to the presidency and his troubled terms in office as a lens to understand the social, economic, and cultural changes in America during the 1960s and 1970s.

13. Hart et al., *Political Keywords,* 1; Leslie Stahl, "Nursing Shortage," *60 Minutes,* June 9, 2002.

14. Roderick P. Hart and Susan Daughton, *Modern Rhetorical Criticism,* 155–57.

15. Rebecca Klatch, "Of Meanings and Masters: Political Symbolism and Symbolic Action," 138, 145.

16. Harold M. Schmeck, "What the Government Can and Cannot Do," *New York Times,* July 13, 1969, E6; "Clinton's Health Plan: Taking His Message to Congress," *New York Times,* September 23, 1993, A25; John Kerry, "Health Care for All Americans."

17. Dan Rather, "Part 1: Your Money or Your Life," *48 Hours,* May 26, 1993.

18. Hart et al., *Political Keywords;* Robin Toner and Sheryl Gay Stolberg, "Decade After Health Care Crisis, Soaring Costs Bring New Strains," *New York Times,* August 11, 2002; Mike Allen and Amy Goldstein, "Bush Urges Malpractice Damage Limits; Plan Includes Goals Sought by Business," *Washington Post,* July 26, 2002, A4; Kelly O'Donnell, "California May Have Found the Solution to Stabilizing Medical Malpractice Insurance Premiums," *NBC Nightly News,* January 3, 2003.

19. Matt Lauer, *Today,* August 7, 2003; Katherine S. Mangan, "The Malpractice Menace."

20. Langston, *With Reverence and Contempt,* 4; Edelman, *Constructing the Political Spectacle,* 31.

21. This definition, provided by I. A. Richards (*The Philosophy of Rhetoric,* 1936), appears in Richard Ohmann, "In Lieu of a New Rhetoric." See also Hacker, *Wittgenstein,* 9.

22. Dan E. Beauchamp, *Health Care Reform and the Battle for the Body Politic,* 156; David Nye, *Narratives and Spaces: Technology and the Construction of American Culture,* 3.

23. Sanford Schram and Philip Neisser, introduction to *Tales of the State: Narrative in Contemporary U.S. Politics and Public Policy,* x.

24. Walter Fisher, *Human Communication as Narration,* 64, 88.

25. Deborah Stone, *Policy Paradox: The Art of Political Decision Making,* 138.

26. Fisher, *Human Communication as Narration,* 76.

27. Kuklick, *Good Ruler,* 28–30.

TWO   The Cost Crisis

1. Mary Wooley and Stacie Propst, "Public Attitudes and Perceptions About Health-Related Research."

2. Peter Jennings and Dean Reynolds, "Health Care Burden on Strike," *World News Tonight with Peter Jennings,* October 14, 2003; Francis X. Clines, "Reagan Asks Doctors to Support Freeze in Their Medicaid Returns," *New York Times,* June 24, 1983, D14; Paul B. Ginsberg, "Controlling Health Care Costs," 1591; Janet Adamy and Laura Meckler, "Obama Makes Case for Health Care Overhaul," *Wall Street Journal,* July 1, 2009.

3. Constance Matthiessen, "Bordering on Collapse," 32; Jennings and Reynolds, "Health Care Burden on Strike."

4. John Iglehart, "The American Health Care System: Expenditures."

5. Ron Allen, "California Workers on Strike over Health Care Benefits," *NBC Nightly News,* December 13, 2003.

6. Howard Rusk, "Rising Hospital Costs," *New York Times,* February 25, 1968, 51.

7. Victor R. Fuchs, "The Growing Demand for Medical Care," 190; Herman M. Somers and Anne R. Somers, *Doctors, Patients, and Health Insurance;* Ruth S. Hanft, "National Health Expenditures, 1950-65," 9; "Gardiner Deplores Health Costs' Rise," *New York Times,* August 10, 1967, 41.

8. Irving Spiegel, "Kennedy Assails Health Plans, Will Urge Congressional Study," *New York Times,* November 20, 1967; Rusk, "Rising Hospital Costs"; Howard Rusk, "Costs of Health Care," *New York Times,* May 12, 1968, 64; Robert H. Phelps, "Senate to Widen Inquiries on Rising Health Care Costs," *New York Times,* January 15, 1968, 18.

9. "Text of White House Report on Health Care Needs," *New York Times,* July 11, 1969, 40; John Hamilton, "Grave Crisis over Rising Costs," *New York Times,* October 26, 1969, E6.

10. "Excerpts from the President's Message Urging 'a New National Health Strategy,'" *New York Times,* February 19, 1971, 16; Harry Schwartz, "An Rx for 'Massive Crisis' in Health Care," *New York Times,* February 21, 1971, E1; Senator Richard Schweiker, "Examination of the Health Care Crisis in America," Hearings Before the Subcommittee on Health, Committee on Labor and Public Welfare, US Senate, 92nd Cong., 1st sess., February 22, 1971, 5.

11. "Americans Said to Spend Ninth of Income on Health," *New York Times,* March 30, 1976, 34; Richard Lyons, "Carter and Health Care Costs," *New York Times,* April 30, 1977, 12; Richard D. Lyons, "Law for Tough Controls on Hospital Charges," *New York Times,* April 26, 1977, 1; "Starting over on High Medical Costs," *New York Times,* November 21, 1979, A18; Tom Wicker, "The National Health," *New York Times,* April 9, 1978; "Mondale Warns on Rise in Cost of Hospital Care," *New York Times,* November 14, 1979, B6; Philip Shabecoff, "Runaway Medical Costs Forcing Hospitals to Reconsider Methods," *New York Times,* May 12, 1978, 15.

12. Bernard Weintraub, "Health Cost Curb Asked by Mondale," *New York Times,* January 7, 1984, 8; Robert Pear, "Increase in Cost of Health Care Drops to 6.3%," *New York Times,* July 10, 1984, A1.

13. Charles Osgood, "Americans Concerned About Rising Health Care Costs," *CBS*

Morning News, September 26, 1991; Bob Arnot, "How America's Health Care Costs Are Spiraling Upward," *CBS This Morning,* December 9, 1991.

14. Martin Tolchin, "Panel Says Broad Health Care Would Cost $86 Billion a Year," *New York Times,* March 3, 1990, 9; Bob Kerrey, "Remarks to the National Newspaper Association Government Affairs Conference"; Laurence Kotlikoff, *The Healthcare Fix,* 1; Greg Hitt and Laura Meckler, "Democrats Ready to Deal on Health," *Wall Street Journal,* July 21, 2009; Janet Adamy, "Health Groups Detail Plans to Reduce Costs," *Wall Street Journal,* June 2, 2009.

15. Fareed Zakaria, "America's Fatal Flaw"; "Opening Bids on Health Care Contain Good Ideas, Big Costs," *USA Today,* July 16, 2009, A8; Olympia Snowe, interview with Matt Lauer, *Today,* October 14, 2009.

16. Nancy Hicks, "Soaring Health Insurance Costs Debated at Auto Talks," *New York Times,* August 22, 1976, 24.

17. William K. Stevens, "High Medical Costs Under Attack as Drain on the Nation's Economy," *New York Times,* March 28, 1982, 50; Joseph Califano, "U.S. Must Discipline Health-Care Market," *New York Times,* May 6, 1984, 226; Mark McEwen and John Stehr, "A Look at the Rising Cost of Health Insurance," *CBS This Morning,* December 11, 1991.

18. Bob Kerrey, "How to Control Health Care Costs," *New York Times,* August 19, 1991, A15; Robert Pear, "Kerrey's Companies Provide Few with Medical Coverage," *New York Times,* December 28, 1991, 1; Stephen Aug, *Business World* (ABC News), February 2, 1992; William J. Clinton, "Address Before a Joint Session of Congress."

19. "Detroit's Health Care Tar Pit," *Wall Street Journal,* July 18, 2003, A8; Milt Freudenheim, "Medical Costs Likely to Slow, but Not Soon," *New York Times,* December 6, 2004, C16; Lee Hawkins and Joseph White, "GM to Seek Sweeping Cutbacks in Union Health-Care Benefits," *Wall Street Journal,* March 24, 2005, A2; Alan Murray, "Health Care Overhaul: GM CEO Weighs In," *Wall Street Journal,* February 9, 2005, A2; Daniel Gross, "Whose Problem Is Health Care?," *New York Times,* February 8, 2004, BU6; "Rip Van UAW," *Wall Street Journal,* October 19, 2005, A12; Kotlikoff, *The Healthcare Fix,* 8; Barack Obama, "Transcript of Address to the 2009 Annual Meeting of the AMA House of Delegates."

20. Robin Toner and Sheryl Gay Stolberg, "Decade After Health Care Crisis, Soaring Costs Bring New Strains," *New York Times,* August 11, 2002; Diane Lewis, "Business Group Sounds Health Insurance Warning," *Boston Globe,* April 18, 2002, C1; Jackie Judd, "Health Insurance Problems," *World News Tonight with Peter Jennings,* April 22, 2003; Vanessa Fuhrmans, "Health Care Costs for Companies, Employees Surge," *Wall Street Journal,* September 10, 2004, A2.

21. Kris Hudson, "Wal-Mart CEO Urges Broader Health Care Cure," *Wall Street Journal,* February 27, 2006; "Transcript of the Second Presidential Debate," *Wall Street Journal,* October 14, 2008; Barack Obama, *Weekly Radio Address.*

22. Max Baucus, "The Senate Is Ready to Act on Health Care," *Wall Street Journal,* September 16, 2009; Gary Locke, "Fixing Health Care Is Good for Business," *Wall Street Journal,* August 26, 2009.

23. William J. Clinton, "Letter to Congressional Leaders"; Milt Freudenheim, "Cost

of Insuring Workers' Health Increases 11.2%," *New York Times,* September 10, 2004, C1; Barack Obama, *Weekly Radio Address;* Obama, "Transcript of Address to the AMA-House of Delegates."

24. Kissick, "Health Policy Directions for the 1970s," 1345; Somers and Somers, *Doctors, Patients and Health Insurance,* 362–63, 492.

25. Rusk, "Rising Hospital Costs"; David J. Rothman, *Beginnings Count: The Technological Imperative in American Health Care,* 4.

26. Richard Nixon, "Transcript of the President's State of the Union Address to the Joint Session of Congress," *New York Times,* January 23, 1971, 12.

27. David Mechanic, "Some Dilemmas in Health Care Policy."

28. William Schwartz, *Life Without Disease: The Pursuit of Medical Utopia;* Charles Bertrand, "Medical Costs Worth Price," *New York Times,* August 3, 1980, WC18.

29. "Starting over on High Medical Costs"; Bertrand, "Medical Costs Worth Price."

30. Irwin Seltzer, "Pricing Health Care: There Is No Health Care Crisis," *Wall Street Journal,* January 24, 1994; Charles Morris, *Too Much of a Good Thing? Why Health Care Spending Won't Make Us Sick,* 3; Steve Lohr, "Health Care Costs Are a Killer, but Maybe That's a Plus," *New York Times,* September 26, 2004, WK5.

31. William Frist, "Health Care in the 21st Century," 268, 271; "NIH Chief: Medicine's Future Is Here," *USA Today,* August 3, 2011, A9.

32. Transcript of *Healthcare Crisis: Who's at Risk?* aired on PBS on November 3, 2000, http://www.pbs.org/healthcarecrisis/transcript.html.

33. Robert J. Blendon and John M. Benson, "Americans' Views on Health Policy: A Fifty-Year Historical Perspective," 38–39; Blendon and Benson, "Understanding How Americans View Health Care Reform," e(13)1–e(13)4.

34. Morris, *Too Much of a Good Thing?;* Wooley and Propst, "Public Attitudes and Perceptions," 1380–81; Robert J. Samuelson, "Obama's Unhealthy Choices."

35. Schwartz, *Life Without Disease,* 16; David Wessel, "Health Care Costs Blamed for Hiring Gap," *Wall Street Journal,* March 11, 2004.

36. Mark McClellan, "Testimony Before the Joint Economic Committee's Hearing on Technology, Innovation, and Health Care Costs," S. Hearing 108-209, 108th Cong., 1st sess., July 9, 2003; Geoffrey Cowley, "The Future of Medicine."

37. Richard G. Frank, "Prescription Drug Prices," 1375; transcript of *Healthcare Crisis: Who's At Risk?*

38. Richard D. Lyon, "Money in Health Is Attracting Many Nonmedical Companies," *New York Times,* March 24, 1968, F1; Robert Cole, "Health Industry Has an Uneasy Feeling," *New York Times,* January 6, 1969, 130.

39. Judith R. Lave and Lester Lave, *The Hospital Construction Act: An Evaluation of the Hill-Burton Program, 1948–1973;* Cole, "Health Industry Has Uneasy Feeling."

40. Thomas J. Lueck, "Health Care Keeps Rank as Job Leader," *New York Times,* May 25, 1993, B1; Iglehart, "American Health Care System," 75.

41. US Department of Labor, Bureau of Labor Statistics, *Occupational Outlook Handbook.*

42. David Bird, "Hospitals Defend Increasing Costs," *New York Times,* June 20, 1976,

35; Steven Roberts, "Hospital Cost Bill Defeat: Elements in the Decision," *New York Times*, November 20, 1979, D15; Robert Reinhold, "Medical Leaders Growing Wary over Reagan Health Care Plans," *New York Times*, February 16, 1981, A12.

43. Thomas Sowell, "Memo to Medical Reformers"; William Safire, "Let's Make a Deal on Health," *New York Times*, May 23, 1994, A15; Elizabeth McCaughey, "No Exit"; Stuart Butler, "Rube Goldberg: Call Your Office," *New York Times*, June 12, 1994, A4, 6.

44. Martin Feldstein, "ObamaCare Is All About Rationing," *Wall Street Journal*, August 18, 2009; Associated Press, "Senate Plows to 1st Vote on Health Care," *USA Today*, December 2, 2009, A8.

45. *Health, United States, 2004*, table 115, http://www.cdc.gov/nchs/data/hus /hus04.pdf (accessed April 17, 2012); "Obama's Health Cost Illusion," *Wall Street Journal*, June 8, 2009; Zakaria, "America's Fatal Flaw"; Daniel Callahan, "Cost Control: Time to Get Serious."

46. Fuchs, "Growing Demand for Medical Care," 192; Mechanic, "Some Dilemmas in Health Care Policy," 3; Wooley and Propst, "Public Attitudes and Perceptions," 1381; Mechanic, "Some Dilemmas in Health Care Policy," 3.

47. G. K. Chesterton, *What's Wrong with the World?*

THREE   The Medical Malpractice Crisis

1. Joie Chen, "Doctors Opting to Practice Without Malpractice Insurance," *CBS Evening News*, November 6, 2004; Jeffrey Kofman, "Doctors on Strike: Health Care Crisis," *World News Tonight with Peter Jennings*, June 18, 2003.

2. Michael J. Halberstam, "The Doctor's New Dilemma—'Will I Be Sued?,'" SM35; David Studdert, Michelle Mello, and Troyen Brennan, "Medical Malpractice," 285; Lawrence Gostin, "A Public Health Approach to Reducing Error," 1743.

3. Randall Bovbjerg, "Medical Malpractice: Folklore, Facts, and the Future"; Michelle Mello, "Managing Malpractice Crises," 414.

4. Lesley Oelsner, "Doctor and Lawyer Cooperation Urged," *New York Times*, August 8, 1975, 19.

5. Lawrence K. Altman, "Malpractice Crisis Overshadows Agenda as A.M.A. Session Opens," *New York Times*, June 15, 1975, 44.

6. Francis X. Clines, "Insurance-Squeezed Doctors Fold Tents," *New York Times*, June 13, 2002, A24; Jeffrey Piccola, "Cap Noneconomic Damages, Attorneys' Fees."

7. Frank Sloan, "State Responses to the Malpractice Insurance 'Crisis' of the 1970s: An Empirical Assessment"; Stephen Shmanske and Tina Stevens, "The Performance of Medical Malpractice Review Panels"; David Margolick, "Medical Malpractice: Role of Lawyers," *New York Times*, February 21, 1985, A16; "Bush Wants Limits on Medical Malpractice Verdicts," *Dow Jones Newswires*, November 16, 2004.

8. Mike Von Fremd, *ABC World News Tonight*, June 30, 1987; Donald J. Palmisano, "Why Your Doctor Might Quit," 50.

9. Wyatt Andrews, "Presidential Candidates' Positions on Medical Malpractice Lawsuits," *CBS Evening News*, November 1, 2004; Obama, "Transcript of Address."

10. US Department of Health, Education, and Welfare, *Medical Malpractice: Report*

of the Secretary's Commission on Medical Malpractice; Nancy Hicks, "H.E.W. Seeks to End 'Crisis' over Medical Malpractice Insurance," *New York Times,* December 28, 1974, 7; "The Malpractice Crisis," *New York Times,* April 4, 1975, 32.

11. James C. Mohr, "American Medical Malpractice Litigation in Historical Perspective," 1733; Joseph F. Sadusk, "Hazardous Fields of Medicine in Relation to Professional Liability," 957.

12. Halberstam, "The Doctor's New Dilemma"; Sara Rosenbaum, "The Impact of United States Law on Medicine as a Profession"; Andrew Sandor, "The History of Professional Liability Suits in the United States," 460; Richard Anderson, "Defending the Practice of Medicine," 1174.

13. John Chancellor and Robert Hagar presented an extended segment on malpractice insurance on the *NBC Nightly News* on January 7, 1975, and Walter Cronkite and Robert Schakne featured rising malpractice rates' effect on doctors' bills on the *CBS Evening News* on January 23, 1975.

14. Lester Sobel, ed., "Malpractice Dilemma," 173. Summaries of television news coverage of the malpractice crisis were obtained from the Vanderbilt Television News Archive. Abstracts of each news story can be found online at http://tvnews .vanderbilt.edu/ (accessed December 26, 2011).

15. "Malpractice Crisis: How It's Hurting Medical Care," *U.S. News and World Report,* May 26, 1975, 32; John Chancellor, Bob Flick, and Fred Briggs, "Malpractice Insurance Controversy," *NBC Nightly News,* May 1, 1975.

16. "Doctors on Coast Meet on Reforms," *New York Times,* June 2, 1975, 53; Lacey Fosburgh, "Physician Strike May Be Widened," *New York Times,* May 25, 1975, 108.

17. "Doctors Press Slowdowns in 2 States," *New York Times,* June 4, 1975, 85; Sobel, "Malpractice Dilemma'; Paul Montgomery, "Doctors Planning Treatment Curbs in Insurance Fight," *New York Times,* April 28, 1975.

18. Jeffrey Kofman, "Doctors in Florida Are Protesting Rising Costs in Malpractice Insurance," *World News Tonight Sunday,* July 21, 2002; Kofman, "Doctors on Strike"; Tom Brokaw, "West Virginia Surgeons Protest Ever Higher Price of Buying Medical Malpractice Insurance," *NBC Nightly News,* January 2, 2003; Iver Peterson, "New Jersey Doctors Hold Back Services in Protest," *New York Times,* February 4, 2003.

19. Peter Jennings and Joe Spencer, *ABC World News Tonight,* October 22, 1985; Diane Sawyer, *Good Morning America,* April 29, 2003; Randall Pinkston, "More Doctors Claiming Malpractice Insurance Costs Are Driving Them Out of Business," *CBS Evening News,* February 23, 2003.

20. Neil A. Lewis, "Senate Rejects Limit on Compensation for Pain," *New York Times,* May 3, 1995, A19.

21. Halberstam, "The Doctor's New Dilemma," SM8; Glen O. Robinson, "The Medical Malpractice Crisis of the 1970s: A Retrospective"; Hicks, "H.E.W. Seeks to End 'Crisis'"; Altman, "Malpractice Crisis Overshadows Agenda"; Sobel, "Malpractice Dilemma."

22. Michelle Mello, David Studdert, and Troyen Brennan, "The New Medical Malpractice Crisis," 2281.

23. Lawrence K. Altman, "Surgeon Group Proposes Reforms to Reduce Malprac-

tice Disparities," *New York Times,* December 2, 1976, 26; Joel Brinkley, "A.M.A. Study Finds Big Rise in Claims for Malpractice," *New York Times,* January 17, 1985, A1.

24. Philip K. Howard, "There Is No 'Right to Sue,'" *Wall Street Journal,* July 31, 2002, A14; George W. Bush, "Remarks at High Point University in High Point, North Carolina," 1254; Joie Chen, "Debate Rages over Proposed Caps on Pain and Suffering Awards in Medical Malpractice Suits," *CBS Evening News,* April 22, 2003; Kofman, "Doctors in Florida"; Chen, "Doctors Opting to Practice Without Malpractice Insurance."

25. Mike Allen and Amy Goldstein, "Bush Urges Malpractice Damage Limits; Plan Includes Goals Sought by Business," *Washington Post,* July 26, 2002, A4; Jay Schadler, *ABC World News Tonight,* May 13, 1985; Joe Spencer, *ABC World News Tonight,* October 22, 1985.

26. Patricia Danzon, "The Frequency and Severity of Medical Malpractice Claims," 118; Edward Gargan, "Doctors and Insurers Press for Limits on Malpractice Awards," *New York Times,* February 21, 1983, B4; Richard Perez-Pena, "Hospitals Fearing Malpractice Crisis," *New York Times,* June 3, 2003, A1; Anderson, "Defending the Practice of Medicine," 1174.

27. Bob Flick's report on malpractice on the *NBC Nightly News* on May 1, 1975, and Dick Shoemaker's segment on the *ABC Evening News* on May 28, 1975, provide examples of how the strike affected patient care. "Creeping Up on Malpractice Reform," *New York Times,* June 29, 1985, 24; Peter Jennings and Mike Von Fremd, *ABC World News Tonight,* January 16, 1987.

28. Mike Von Fremd, *ABC World News Tonight,* June 30, 1987; Michael Myers, "Will Amendment 10 Benefit Florida Residents? Yes," *St. Petersburg Times,* October 22, 1988, 2.

29. Associated Press, "Docs Skip Work to Protest Insurance Costs," *New York Times,* January 28, 2003; Rene Syler, "Dr. Greg Saracco and Wheeling Hospital CEO Dr. Donald Hofreuter Discuss the Medical Crisis Facing West Virginia," *CBS Early Show,* January 2, 2003; Mangan, "The Malpractice Menace," A16; Tom Brokaw, "Doctors, Unable to Afford Rising Malpractice Premiums," *NBC Nightly News,* April 21, 2004.

30. Andrew Malcolm, "Fear of Malpractice Suits Spurring Some Doctors to Leave Obstetrics," *New York Times,* February 12, 1985, A1; Orrin Hatch, "The Medical Malpractice Crisis: Physicians' Concern over Future Liability Costs Is Adversely Affecting Access to Health Care for All Americans"; Francis X. Clines, "Insurance Squeezed Doctors Fold Their Tents," *New York Times,* June 13, 2002, A24; Daniel Eisenberg and Maggie Sieger, "The Doctor Won't See You Now"; Rob Stein, "Critical Condition: Skyrocketing Malpractice Insurance Rates Have Begun to Hurt Patients as Well as Doctors," *Washington Post National Weekly Edition,* January 13–19, 2003, 29.

31. See Roy Neal's reports on the malpractice crisis in Southern California aired on the *NBC Evening News* on December 10, 1975, and December 14, 1975. The *CBS Evening News* broadcast a similar story on the situation in Southern California on January 1, 1976. Mike Von Fremd, *ABC World News Tonight,* June 30, 1987; Eisenberg and Sieger, "The Doctor Won't See You Now"; Charles Gibson, "Doctors Closing Down Practices Due to High Costs of Malpractice Insurance," *ABC World News Tonight,* July 23, 2002.

32. Halberstam, "The Doctor's New Dilemma"; "Malpractice Crisis: How It's Hurting Medical Care"; Kandy G. Webb, "Recent Medical Malpractice Legislation: A First Checkup," 655.

33. David A. Hyman and Charles Silver, "Believing Six Improbable Things: Medical Malpractice and 'Legal Fear'"; Halberstam, "The Doctor's New Dilemma," SM8–9; Hicks, "H.E.W. Seeks End to 'Crisis.'"

34. Sobel, "Malpractice Dilemma," 170.

35. Milt Freudenheim, "Dealing in Myths on Malpractice," *New York Times*, October 13, 1992, D2; William J. Clinton, "Remarks in the ABC News *Nightline* Town Meeting in Tampa, Florida," 1863.

36. Bush, "Remarks at High Point University," 1251; Allen and Goldstein, "Bush Urges Malpractice Damage Limits"; John McCain, "Remarks at a Town Hall Meeting in Sun City, Arizona"; Mitch McConnell, remarks on the Senate floor, October 20, 2009.

37. Jay Schadler, *ABC World News Tonight*, May 13, 1985; Bob Arnot, "How to Deal with Spiraling Health Care Costs," *CBS This Morning*, December 12, 1991; David Studdert et al., "Defensive Medicine Among High-Risk Specialist Physicians in a Volatile Malpractice Environment."

38. Harvey Wachsman, letter to the editor, *New York Times*, September 9, 1983, A18.

39. "Lawyers Assail Striking Doctors," *New York Times*, May 14, 1975, 36; "Progressive Doctors, Not Incompetents, the Most Often Sued, Hearing Is Told," *New York Times*, October 25, 1975, 63; Fred Queller, "Legal Perspectives on New York's Medical Malpractice Reform," *New York Times*, July 10, 1985, A22; Mike Von Fremd, *ABC World News Tonight*, January 16, 1987.

40. Jane Robelot, "Distinguishing Between Medical Mistakes and Medical Malpractice," *CBS This Morning*, October 9, 1997.

41. During the fourth season of *ER*, the episodes "Something New" and "Good Touch, Bad Touch," aired in 1997, dedicated considerable attention to malpractice issues. In the first episode, Dr. Greene was served with a wrongful-death suit by the Law family; three weeks later, he participated in an acrimonious deposition with the family's lawyer.

42. See the episode "Infected" from season 3 of *The Practice*, in which the firm's lawyers work on a wrongful-death suit for a woman who died after routine cosmetic surgery, and "Race Ipsa Loquitor" from season 4, when a woman sues after her husband dies during a liposuction procedure.

43. See the interview with Chris Murphy, *ABC Evening News*, June 16, 1975, and the special reports by Mike Jackson, *NBC Nightly News*, June 23–24, 1975.

44. Dan Rather, "Medical Malpractice Sends Two to Grave; Accidents Becoming More of an Everyday Occurrence," *CBS Evening News*, March 16, 1995; Robelot, "Distinguishing Between Medical Mistakes and Medical Malpractice."

45. Chen, "Debate Rages over Proposed Caps on Pain and Suffering Awards"; Diane Sawyer, "Battling Insurance Caps: One Victim's Point of View," *Good Morning America*, March 12, 2003.

46. "Lawyers Assail Striking Doctors," *New York Times*, May 14, 1975, 36; Ronald Sullivan, "Cuomo Offers Plan to Cut Malpractice Costs," *New York Times*, April 4, 1985, B6; David Bird, "Malpractice Insurance: A Crisis in Health Care," *New York Times*, January

19, 1975, 1; "Progressive Doctors, Not Incompetents, the Most Often Sued"; Mike Von Fremd, *ABC World News Tonight,* June 30, 1987.

47. Stuart Taylor, "Lawyers Deny Crisis in Medical Malpractice Insurance," *New York Times,* March 7, 1985, A16; Nicolas Kristof, "Insurance Woes Spur Many States to Amend Law on Liability Suits," *New York Times,* March 31, 1986, A1; Katharine Seelye, "Playing the Tort Card," *New York Times,* September 18, 2009.

48. Richard Earle, "Will Amendment 10 Benefit Florida Residents? No," *St. Petersburg Times,* October 22, 1988, 2; Clines, "Insurance-Squeezed Doctors Fold Their Tents," A24.

49. Stanley Rosenblatt, "In His Own Words"; Martin Tolchin, "Concern over the Cost of Malpractice Liability," *New York Times,* November 5, 1989, E4; David Margolick, "Role of Lawyers," *New York Times,* February 21, 1985, A16.

50. Charlayne Hunter, "Trial Lawyers Assail Medical Society," *New York Times,* May 25, 1976, 32; Fred Queller, "Making the Case for Trial Lawyers," *New York Times,* November 10, 1984, 22; Steve Lohr, "Bush's Next Target: Malpractice Lawyers," *New York Times,* February 27, 2005.

51. Hillary Rodham Clinton and Barack Obama, "Making Patient Safety the Centerpiece of Medical Liability Reform," 2207.

52. Halberstam, "The Doctor's New Dilemma."

53. Lucian Leape et al., "Promoting Patient Safety by Preventing Medical Error," 1444; Gostin, "Public Health Approach," 1742.

54. Rideout, *Television as a Health Educator;* Laura Keaney, "Examining Medical Error: Causes, Consequences, and Checklists"; Atul Gawande, *The Checklist Manifesto,* 103; Institute of Medicine, *To Err Is Human: Building a Safer Health Care System—Report Brief,* 2.

55. Rita Rubin, "Dennis Quaid Takes Aim at Health Care Mistakes," *USA Today,* April 12, 2010.

56. James T. Reason, "Human Error: Models and Management," 770; Brian Liang, "Risks of Reporting Sentinel Events"; Gostin, "Public Health Approach."

57. American Hospital Association, "Prescriptions for Reform: Patient Safety—a Key Ingredient of Any Reform," *Wall Street Journal,* November 20, 2009, A27.

58. Atul Gawande, *Complications;* Stephen C. Schoenbaum and Randall Bovbjerg, "Malpractice Reform Must Include Steps to Prevent Medical Injury."

59. Gawande, *The Checklist Manifesto.*

60. Keaney, "Examining Medical Error."

61. John Hill, "The Power of 'I'm Sorry,'" *Providence Sunday Journal,* December 6, 2009, 1, 10.

62. Michelle Mello and Thomas Gallagher, "Malpractice Reform: Opportunities for Leadership by Health Care Institutions and Liability Insurers," 1353.

63. Ryan Boyle, "A Red Moon over the Mall: The Sputnik Panic and Domestic America"; Dennis Quaid, Julie Thao, and Charles Denham, "Story Power: The Secret Weapon," 5.

FOUR   The Nurse Staffing Crisis

1. See Bobbi Kimball and Edward O'Neil, "The Evolution of a Crisis: Nursing in America"; Robert Steinbrook, "Nursing in the Crossfire"; Howard Berliner and Eli Ginsberg, "Why This Nursing Shortage Is Different."

2. Quoted in Milan Korcok, "'Perfect Storm' Brewing in US Because of Nursing Shortage."

3. Tony Dokupil, "When Nurses Strike in New York"; Alice Gomstyn, "Thousands of Nurses Strike in Minnesota," *ABC News,* June 10, 2010; Associated Press, "12,000 Minnesota Nurses Launch One Day Strike," CBS News.com, June 10, 2010; Maura Lerner, "Deal Was 'a Win' for Both Sides," *Minneapolis Star-Tribune,* July 2, 2010.

4. Hacker, *Wittgenstein,* 13; Roger Jones, "Analytic Philosophy."

5. Letter to the editor, *New York Times,* December 12, 1945, 25; "Nurses Needed," *New York Times,* March 14, 1948, E8; Harold Faber, "Shortage of Nurses Found a Peril to Health of Nation," *New York Times,* March 3, 1952, 1; "Shortage of Nurses Seen," *New York Times,* November 16, 1947, 4; letter to the editor, *New York Times,* September 30, 1947, C24.

6. Richard Steckel, "Hospitals and Beds, by Type of Hospital: 1946–1997"; Bess Furman, "Need for Nurses Put to Congress," *New York Times,* May 22, 1955, 79; "Hospitals Report Nurse Shortage," *New York Times,* November 28, 1954, 125.

7. Lacey Fosburgh, "Nurses on Coast Still on Strike," *New York Times,* June 12, 1974, 12; "Emergency Care Halted by Nurses Striking on Coast," *New York Times,* June 20, 1974, 25; Tom Brokaw, "Nurse Strike Seriously Affects San Francisco Bay Area," *NBC Nightly News,* June 19, 1974; Harry Reasoner, "Striking Nurses in San Francisco Pull Intensive Care Unit Nurses Off Posts in Effort to Reach Some Settlement," *ABC Evening News,* June 20, 1974; Harry Reasoner, "San Francisco Nurses Strike Worsens," *ABCEvening News,* June 21, 1974; "Accord Reached in Nurses Strike," *New York Times,* June 27, 1974, 14; "Nurses in California End a 3-Week Strike with 11% Pay Raises," *New York Times,* June 29, 1974, 59.

8. Max Robinson, *ABC World News Tonight,* October 8, 1981; Steven Geer, *ABC World News Tonight,* October 5, 1981.

9. Milt Freudenheim, "Nursing Shortage Is Costing Billions," *New York Times,* May 31, 1988, D2; Sally Reed, "Streamlining Education of New Nurses," *New York Times,* October 11, 1987, A1; Tamar Lewin, "Sudden Nurse Shortage Threatens Hospital Care," *New York Times,* July 7, 1987, A1.

10. Joint Commission on the Accreditation of Healthcare Organizations, *Health Care at the Crossroads: Strategies for Addressing the Evolving Nursing Crisis,* 5.

11. "This Nursing Shortage Is Different," *New York Times,* December 20, 1988, A26.

12. Tom Brokaw and Robert Bazell, "Shortage of Qualified Nurses Becoming Major US Problem," *NBC Nightly News,* February 13, 2001; Bob Schieffer, "Nursing Shortage May Be Putting Lives at Risk," *CBS Evening News,* May 24, 2006; Lester Holt and Robert Bazell, "Shortage of Nurses Around the Country Could Affect Quality of Health Care," *NBC Nightly News,* July 6, 2007.

13. "Report Cites Danger in Nurse Shortage," *New York Times,* September 13, 1948,

16; letter to the editor, *New York Times,* July 26, 1960, 28; Foster Hailey, "Nursing Shortage Still Acute Here," *New York Times,* July 4, 1960, 1.

14. William Knaus, "Nurses Can No Longer Be Taken for Granted," *New York Times,* November 24, 1980, A27; Ronald Sullivan, "Conditions at Lincoln Hospital Described as Worse than on Battlefield," *New York Times,* December 5, 1976, 76.

15. Lawrence K. Altman, "New Demands Straining City's Hospitals," *New York Times,* October 7, 1986, B1; Robert MacNeil and Elizabeth Brackett, "Care Crisis," *The MacNeil/Lehrer NewsHour,* July 27, 1988.

16. Sanjay Gupta, "Special Report: U.S. Nursing Shortage 'Going into Crisis,'" *CNN Medical News,* May 7, 2001; Dianne Anderson, "Testimony Before the US Senate Subcommittee on Aging, Committee on Health, Education, Labor, and Pensions," February 13, 2001; Leslie Stahl, "Nursing Shortage in Critical Stage," *CBS News,* January 17, 2003; Hannah Storm and Hattie Kauffman, "Edith Rodriguez Dies After Being Left in ER Lobby," *CBS Early Show,* June 14, 2007; Ann Curry and Nancy Synderman, "ER Overburdened, Understaffed," *NBC Nightly News,* October 9, 2007.

17. Harold Faber, "Shortage of Nurses Found a Peril to Health of Nation," *New York Times,* March 3, 1952, 12.

18. Diana Olick and Thalia Assuras, "Nationwide Nursing Shortage Affecting Many Hospitals," *CBS Morning News,* December 29, 2000; Charles Osgood, "Nursing Shortage Getting Critical," *CBS News: The Osgood File,* October 23, 2002; Gail Collins, "Nursing a Shortage," *New York Times,* April 13, 2001, A17.

19. Bobbi Kimball and Edward O'Neil, *Health Care's Human Crisis: The American Nursing Shortage;* Joint Commission on the Accreditation of Healthcare Organizations, *Health Care at the Crossroads,* 5.

20. Sanjay Gupta, "Nurses Face Problems," *CNN: Your Health,* May 12, 2001; Joann Loviglio, "Nurses Desert Profession; Men Leave at Twice the Rate of Women," *Washington Post,* October 20, 2002, A21; Arlene Weintraub, "Nursing: On the Critical List."

21. Tom Brokaw and Robert Bazell, "Nurse Shortages and Long Work Shifts Create Dangerous Future Prospects for Patients," *NBC Nightly News,* November 7, 2003; Anne Thompson, "Nationwide Nursing and Nursing Instructor Shortages," *Today,* September 5, 2003; Sara Corbett, "The Last Shift."

22. "For Want of a Nurse," *New York Times,* May 27, 2006, A12.

23. Harold Faber, "Nurse Lack Acute at City Hospitals," *New York Times,* March 4, 1952, 16; Ronald Sullivan, "Nurse Scarcity Forces Cut in Care in New York Municipal Hospitals," *New York Times,* August 6, 1981, A1.

24. George Strait, *ABC World News Tonight,* May 9, 1989; Luz Ramos, "Caring Till It Hurts," *New York Times,* May 27, 2001, NJ15; Charles Gibson and Michelle Norris, "Nursing Shortage," *Good Morning America,* August 8, 2002; Robert Bazell, "Nurse Shortages and Long Work Shifts Create Dangerous Future Prospects for Patients," *NBC Nightly News,* November 7, 2003.

25. Sullivan, "Nurse Scarcity," A1; Steven Geer, *ABC World News Tonight,* October 5, 1981; Altman, "New Demands," B1; Michael Berens, "Nursing Mistakes Kill, Injure Thousands," *Chicago Tribune,* September 10, 2000; Weintraub, "Nursing."

26. Ramos, "Caring Till It Hurts"; Paul Duke, "If ER Nurses Crash, Will Patients Fol-

low?"; John Blanton, "Care and Chaos on the Night Nursing Shift," *Wall Street Journal,* April 24, 2007.

27. Sullivan, "Conditions at Lincoln Hospital"; Sheryl Gay Stolberg, "Patient Deaths Tied to Lack of Nurses," *New York Times,* August 8, 2002, A18; Laura Johannes, "Serious Health Risk Posed by Lack of Nurses," *Wall Street Journal,* May 30, 2002, D1; John Seigenthaler, "Study Shows Shortage of Nurses Contributes to Hospital Errors," *NBC Nightly News,* August 10, 2002; Robert Bazell, "In Depth," *NBC Nightly News,* November 7, 2003; George Lewis, "Severe Nursing Shortage Having Direct, Sometimes Deadly Impact on Patients and Families," *NBC Nightly News,* April 5, 2002; Nancy Synderman, "Dr. Nancy Synderman Discusses New Study's Findings," *Today,* April 7, 2008.

28. Thalia Assuras, "Eye on America," *CBS Evening News,* December 28, 2000; Sanjay Gupta, "Nursing Shortage Continues to Grow," *CNN: Live Today,* May 9, 2001; Storm and Kauffman, "Edith Rodriguez Dies"; Synderman, "Dr. Nancy Synderman Discusses New Study's Findings."

29. Trust for America's Health, "Nursing Shortage Estimates (2010)"; Lawrence R. Jacobs, "1994 All Over Again? Public Opinion and Health Care," 1883.

30. "Nurse Shortage Seen," *New York Times,* September 6, 1957, 34; Faber, "Nurse Lack Acute at City Hospitals"; Emma Harrison, "Nursing Shortage May Be on Wane," *New York Times,* August 26, 1956, 79; Geoffrey Pond, "City's Hospitals Short of Nurses," *New York Times,* September 27, 1959, 54; Emma Harrison, "Low Pay Is Scored in City Hospitals," *New York Times,* April 15, 1960, 14; Leonard Engel, "The Ills of 'Maintown' Hospital," *New York Times Magazine,* November 26, 1961, SM43.

31. Kenneth Arrow and William Capron, "Dynamic Shortages and Price Rises: The Engineer-Scientist Case"; Conor Dougherty, "Slowdown's Side Effect: More Nurses," *Wall Street Journal,* May 7, 2008, D1.

32. American Nurses Association, "Effects of the Nursing Shortage," http://ana.nursingworld.org/MainMenuCategories/ThePracticeofProfessionalNursing/workforce/NurseShortageStaffing/NursingShortage/Effects.aspx (accessed April 17, 2012).

33. Bridget Kuehn, "No End in Sight to Nursing Shortage," 1623.

34. Suzanne Gordon, "What Nurses Stand For"; Suzanne Gordon and Bernice Buresh, "Doc Hollywood."

35. Sandra Boodman, "Nurses Protest Their Depiction on TV's *ER,*" *Providence Journal,* December 2003, F1; "The Nursing Shortage and Its Impact on America's Health Care Delivery System," hearings held before the US Senate Subcommittee on Aging, Committee on Health, Education, Labor, and Pensions, February 13, 2001, 4.

36. Carolyn Hope Smeltzer, Frances Vlasses, and Connie Robinson, "'If We Only Had a Nurse' . . . Historical View of a Nurse Shortage."

37. Karen Donelan et al., "Awareness and Perceptions of the Johnson and Johnson Campaign for Nursing's Future: Views from Nursing Students, RNs, and CNOs"; Smeltzer, Vlasses, and Robinson, "'If We Only Had a Nurse'"; Michael M. O'Connor, "The Role of the Television Drama ER in Medical Student Life: Entertainment or Socialization?"

FIVE   **The Health Insurance Crisis**

1. Hendrick Hertzberg, "Electoral Dissonance"; John Iglehart, "Historic Passage: Reform at Last"; Kaiser Family Foundation, *Kaiser Health Tracking Poll: December 2010;* "The Repeal Vote," *Wall Street Journal,* January 20, 2011; Atul Gawande, "Now What?"

2. Len Nichols, "Be Not Afraid," e30(1); "Prepared Text of Obama's Speech on Health Care," *Wall Street Journal,* September 10, 2009; Hendrick Hertzberg, "Lies"; Jonathan Oberlander, "Beyond Repeal: The Future of Health Care Reform."

3. Susan Page and Kelly Kennedy, "U.S. Split on Repeal of Health Care Law," *USA Today,* January 7, 2011, A1; Martin Tolchin, "Panel Says Broad Health Care Would Cost $86 Billion a Year," *New York Times,* March 3, 1990, 9.

4. Denby, "Calculating Rhythm," 90; David Blumenthal, "Health Care Reform at the Close of the 20th Century."

5. "Text of White House Report on Health Care Needs," *New York Times,* July 11, 1969, 40; Harold M. Schmeck, "Fight to Improve Health Care Set," *New York Times,* January 21, 1969, 50.

6. Senator Edward M. Kennedy, "Examination of the Health Care Crisis in America," hearings before the US Senate Subcommittee on Health, Committee on Labor and Public Welfare, 92nd Cong., 1st sess., February 22, 1971, 1; Roger Egeberg, "Health Care Faces Severest Demands," *New York Times,* January 12, 1970, 87; Jacqueline Adams, *Bitter Medicine* (CBS News), May 26, 1993.

7. Carmen DeNavas-Walt, Bernadette D. Proctor, and Cheryl Hill Lee, US Census Bureau, *Current Population Reports, P60-231, Income, Poverty, and Health Insurance Coverage in the United States: 2005,* table C-1; George Lundberg, "National Health Care Reform: An Aura of Inevitability Is upon Us"; Harry Smith, *CBS This Morning,* January 23, 1992.

8. Hillary Clinton, "Remarks on American Health Choices Plan"; Judd Gregg, "Don't Silence the Minority," *USA Today,* March 18, 2010, A10.

9. John McCain, "Text of McCain Speech on Health Care," *Wall Street Journal,* October 11, 2007.

10. Karl Rove, "Republicans Can Win on Health Care," *Wall Street Journal,* September 18, 2007, A15; Hendrick Hertzberg, "Ghostbusters," 38.

11. Michael Crichton, "The High Cost of Cure"; Harry Schwartz, "A Plan for When Medical Disaster Strikes," *New York Times,* December 13, 1970, 200; Edward M. Kennedy, *In Critical Condition: The Crisis in America's Health Care,* 25.

12. Bob Arnot, "How America's Health Care Costs Are Spiraling Upward," *CBS This Morning,* December 9, 1991; Lawrence R. Jacobs, Robert Shapiro, and Eli Shulman, "Medical Care in the United States: An Update."

13. Michael Wines and Robert Pear, "President Finds Benefits in Defeat on Health Care," *New York Times,* July 30, 1996, A1; William J. Clinton, "Address Before a Joint Session of Congress"; "Excerpts from Opening Statements in Health Care Debate," *New York Times,* August 10, 1994.

14. "Transcript of 1992 Vice Presidential Debate," *New York Times,* October 14, 1992, A20.

15. William J. Clinton, "Address Before a Joint Session of the Congress on the State of the Union."

16. American Medical Association, "VoiceForTheUninsured.org."

17. H. Clinton, "Remarks on American Health Choices Plan"; Barack Obama, "Cutting Costs and Covering America: A 21st Century Health Care System"; McCain, "Text of McCain Speech on Health Care."

18. "Yes, There Is a Health Crisis," editorial, *New York Times,* January 30, 1994, E16; Mortimer Zuckerman, "America's High Anxiety."

19. Charles Gibson, *Good Morning America,* October 20, 2003; Wyatt Andrews, "Higher Costs Paid by Uninsured Patients for Hospital Bills," *CBS Early Show;* Diane Sawyer and Kate Snow, *Good Morning America,* February 2, 2005; Robin Roberts and Chris Cuomo, *Good Morning America,* October 16, 2006.

20. Egeberg, "Health Care Faces Severest Demands."

21. Kennedy, *In Critical Condition,* 79.

22. Clinton, "Address Before a Joint Session of Congress."

23. Iver Peterson, "Lost Medical Care for the Jobless: Cost May Be Health or Lives," *New York Times,* March 7, 1983, A1; Jack Smith, *ABC World News Tonight,* January 24, 1993.

24. Bob Hebert, "It's Not Just the Uninsured," *New York Times,* November 17, 2007, 19; Geraldine Ferraro, "How to Mend a Sick System."

25. Dan Rather and Edie Magnus, *CBS Evening News,* September 25, 1991.

26. Jacqueline Adams, *CBS Evening News,* March 3, 1990; Ted Koppel and John McKenzie, *ABC News Nightline,* November 21, 1991; Peter Jennings, *World News Tonight with Peter Jennings,* September 29, 1992.

27. Tom Foley, *CBS News Special Report: State of the Union,* January 28, 1992.

28. Mark McEwen, "A Look at the Rising Cost of Health Insurance," *CBS This Morning,* December 11, 1991; Philip J. Hilts, "Say Ouch: Demands to Fix U.S. Health Care Reach a Crescendo," *New York Times,* May 19, 1991, E1; Tom Brokaw and Jim Avila, *NBC Nightly News,* October 23, 1997; Dan Rather, *CBS Evening News,* July 12, 1999.

29. John M. Broder, Robert Pear, and Milt Freudenheim, "Problem of Lost Health Benefits Is Reaching into the Middle Class," *New York Times,* November 25, 2002, A1, A16; "Health Reform, Piece by Piece," *New York Times,* November 22, 2002, A26; Susan McGinnis, "Survey Finds Health Insurance Premiums Rising Three Times Faster than Workers' Wages," *CBS Morning News,* September 29, 2004.

30. Katie Couric and Matt Lauer, *Today,* October 5, 2004; Peter Jennings, "Breakdown: America's Health Insurance Crisis," *Primetime Live,* December 15, 2005.

31. James A. Morone, *The Democratic Wish,* 438.

32. Albert O. Hirschman, *The Rhetoric of Reaction,* 7.

33. Samuel Huntington, *American Politics: The Promise of Disharmony,* 42; W. H. Lawrence, "Eisenhower Favors Some Aid in Health and Schools by U.S.," *New York Times,* October 9, 1952, 1; Grant McConnell, *Private Power and American Democracy,* 5.

34. Julie Rovner, "'Play or Pay' Gains Momentum as Labor Panel Marks Up Bill"; George Newman, "Parsing the Health Reform Arguments," *Wall Street Journal,* July 1, 2009, A13; Chuck Grassley, "Health Care Reform: A Republican View," 2397–99.

35. Anthony Lewis, "Liberty and Community," *New York Times*, August 23, 1976; Rashi Fein, "Social and Economic Attitudes Shaping American Health Care Policy," 356; Blendon and Benson, "Americans' Views on Health Policy."

36. Russell Baker, "Hazardous to Health," *New York Times*, December 8, 1993, A27; Robert Pear, "Health Insurance Lobbyist Sits Down with White House, but Critical Ads Continue," *New York Times*, January 25, 1994, D21.

37. Pear, "Health Insurance Lobbyist Sits Down with White House."

38. Robert Dole, "Excerpts from the Republicans' Response to the President's Message," *New York Times*, January 26, 1994, A15; Robert Pear, "Diverse Elements Criticize 'Mainstream' Senate Plan," *New York Times*, August 21, 1994, 1, 30.

39. Richard W. Stevenson, "Bush Campaign Unleashes a New Assault on Kerry's Health Care Proposals," *New York Times*, October 13, 2004, A18; George W. Bush, "Health Care Coverage and Drug Costs: The Candidates Speak Out," 1817.

40. "HillaryCare v. Obama," *Wall Street Journal*, January 7, 2008, A12; Mitt Romney, "Where HillaryCare Goes Wrong," *Wall Street Journal*, September 20, 2007, A13.

41. David Jackson, "McCain Would 'Put Families in Charge' of Their Health Care," *USA Today*, June 29, 2008, A4; Laura Meckler, "McCain Pushes a Health Care Plan with Less Regulation," *Wall Street Journal*, April 30, 2008, A6; McCain, "Text of McCain Speech on Health Care."

42. McCain, "Text of McCain Speech on Health Care."

43. John Fritze, "In Run-Up to November, GOP Unveils 'Pledge,'" *USA Today*, September 24, 2010, A9; George Pataki, "Repeal and Replace," *USA Today*, September 13, 2010, A12; David Herszenhom, "Ad Campaigns: The Target? Health Care Law," *New York Times*, September 9, 2010, A20.

44. Mimi Hall, "Health Plan Gets $155B Boost," *USA Today*, July 9, 2009, A6; Mike Enzi, "Public Option Is No Option," *USA Today*, August 19, 2009, A8; "The Worst Bill Ever," *Wall Street Journal*, November 2, 2009.

45. Roger W. Cobb and Charles Elder, *Participation in American Politics*, 39–40.

46. George Allen, "Mandate Is 'Unfair, Harmful,'" *USA Today*, December 14, 2010, A8.

47. Richard Lyons, "Hospital Association Will Study National Health Insurance Plan," *New York Times*, September 9, 1969, 2.

48. Dole, "Excerpts from the Republicans' Response"; American College of Cardiology, "There Is No Debating Our Place in Your Health Care," *New York Times*, June 12, 1994, 5.

49. McCaughey, "No Exit," 21.

50. Thomas Daschle, "Health Care Reform: A Cause Whose Time Has Come," *Washington Post*, March 19, 2009; George Newman, "Parsing the Health Reform Arguments," *Wall Street Journal*, July 1, 2009; John Fritze, "Lawmakers Go Hard Line on Health Care," *USA Today*, September 4, 2009, A4.

51. Betsy McCaughey, "What the Pelosi Health Care Bill Really Says," *Wall Street Journal*, November 9, 2009.

52. Richard Lyons, "Health Aid Plan Scored by H.E.W.," *New York Times*, September 24, 1970, 28; "Excerpts from Platform Approved by G.O.P. Resolutions Panel for the Convention," *New York Times*, August 22, 1972, 35.

53. Robin Toner, "Clinton Facing Reality of Health Care Reform," *New York Times,* May 23, 1993, A14; Robin Toner, "G.O.P. on Health Care: Seeking a Second Opinion," *New York Times,* March 4, 1994, 24.

54. Peggy Noonan, "There Is No New Frontier," *Wall Street Journal,* October 17, 2009, A13; Douglas Holtz-Eakin, "The Coming Deficit Disaster," *Wall Street Journal,* November 20, 2009; Enzi, "Public Option Is No Option."

55. Pataki, "Repeal and Replace"; Employers for a Healthy Economy Coalition, "The Worst Bill Ever," *USA Today,* November 5, 2009, A4.

56. Robin Toner, "Poll Says Public Favors Changes in Health Policy," *New York Times,* April 6, 1993, A1; Jacobs, "1994 All over Again?," 1883; Beatrix Hoffman, "Health Care Reform and Social Movements in the United States," 75.

57. Blendon and Benson, "Americans' Views on Health Policy"; Sydia Saad, "No Increase in Public Pressure for Healthcare Reform"; Humphrey Taylor and Robert Leitman, "Attitudes Towards the United States' Health Care System: Long-Term Trends," 3.

58. George Will, "Word Spill."

59. Charles Siegfried, "The Private Sector," *New York Times,* August 14, 1972, 27; David J. Rothman, "A Century of Failure: Health Care Reform in America," 276; "Governors Hear a Health Debate," *New York Times,* June 4, 1974, 15.

60. Robert Dole, "Is There Really a Health Care Crisis?," *CNN,* December 17, 1993.

61. Dole, "Excerpts from the Republicans' Response"; "Excerpts from Opening Statements in Health Care Debate," *New York Times,* August 10, 1994.

62. Blumenthal, "Health Care Reform," 1916; Hoffman, *The Wages of Sickness;* Anthony Lewis, "Time for a Change," *New York Times,* April 9, 1992, A25.

63. James Mongan and Thomas Lee, "Do We Really Want Broad Access to Health Care?," 1262; Senator Jacob Javits, "Examination of the Health Care Crisis in America," hearings before the US Senate Subcommittee on Health, Committee on Labor and Public Welfare, 92nd Cong., 1st sess., February 22, 1971, 6.

CONCLUSION   A Second Opinion

1. Lawrence Brown, "The Amazing, Non-collapsing U.S. Health Care System: Is Reform Finally at Hand?"

2. George Orwell, "Politics and the English Language"; Hendrick Hertzberg, "Tuesday, and After."

3. George W. Madison et al., "Brief for Petitioners (Minimum Coverage Provision) No. 11-398 Submitted to the Supreme Court of the United States, Re: *Department of Health and Human Services et al. v. State of Florida et al.,*" 2.

4. Kaiser Family Foundation, *Kaiser Health Tracking Poll: December 2011;* Eli Ginsberg, "Health Care Reform: Why So Slow?," 1465; Jonathan Oberlander, "The Politics of Health Reform: Why Do Bad Things Happen to Good Plans?"

5. Blendon and Benson, "Americans' Views on Health Policy," 38.

6. Richard Wolf and John Fritze, "Obama Wants a Health Vote Soon," *USA Today,* March 4, 2010, A1; "Dispute over 'Public Option' Veers into Fantasyland," *USA Today,* August 19, 2009, A8.

7. Evan Thomas and Stuart Taylor Jr., "Fight Club."

8. Morris Fiorina, *Disconnect: The Breakdown of Representation in American Politics;* Alan Abramowitz and Kyle Saunders, "Is Polarization a Myth?"; Morris Fiorina, Samuel Abrams, and Jeremy Pope, "Polarization in the American Public: Misconceptions and Misreadings."

9. Samuel Huntington, "The United States"; James Sundquist, "The Crisis of Competence in Our National Government."

10. Gerald Seib, "Health Debate Isn't About Health," *Wall Street Journal,* August 11, 2009, A2.

11. John Hollander, "Fear Itself," 866.

12. Fisher, *Human Communication as Narration,* 156.

13. Morone, *The Democratic Wish;* Gingrich quoted in Hendrick Hertzberg, "Come Together"; Joe Pitts, "We Need a New Approach," *USA Today,* January 20, 2011, A10.

14. Lawrence Wallack and Regina Lawrence, "Talking About Public Health: Developing America's 'Second Language,'" 567; Beauchamp also offers a communitarian vision for health care reform in *Health Care Reform.*

15. Quoted in Susan Page and David Jackson, "House Republicans Plan Early Vote on Health Care Repeal," *USA Today,* January 3, 2011, A2; Paul Starr, "The Lost Crusade"; Elizabeth Williamson, "Americans Grow Weary of Government Intervention in Marketplace," *Wall Street Journal,* January 19, 2010.

16. Schwartz, *Life Without Disease.*

17. Blendon and Benson, "Americans' Views on Health Policy," 38.

18. Atul Gawande, "Getting There from Here: How Should Obama Reform Health Care?"; Bruce Vladeck, "Universal Health Insurance in the United States: Reflections on the Past, the Present, and the Future," 18.

19. Daniel Yankelovich, "Overcoming Polarization: The New Social Morality," 3; Barack Obama, "Remarks by the President at Signing of Children's Health Insurance Program Legislation"; Uwe Reinhardt, "Wanted: A Clearly Articulated Social Ethic for American Health Care"; Tsung-mei Cheng and Uwe Reinhart, "The Ethics of America's Health Care Debate," 86.

20. Darrell M. West, *Congress and Economic Policymaking;* Nicholas Lemann, "Kennedy Care," 22.

21. Hollander, "Fear Itself," 878; Anthony Lewis, "Time for a Change," *New York Times,* April 9, 1992, 5.

ABC News/Kaiser Family Foundation/USA Today. *Health Care in America 2006 Survey Chartpack.* October 2006. http://www.kff.org/kaiserpolls/upload/7572.pdf.

Abramowitz, Alan, and Kyle Saunders. "Is Polarization a Myth?" *Journal of Politics* 70, no. 2 (2008): 542–55.

Alford, Robert. "The Political Economy of Health Care: Dynamics Without Change." *Politics and Society* 2, no. 2 (1972): 127–64.

American Medical Association. Testimony Before the Committee on Energy and Commerce, Subcommittee on Health, US House of Representatives. February 10, 2005. http://www.ama-assn.org/ama1/pub/upload/mm/363/liabtestimony.pdf.

———. "VoiceForTheUninsured.org." http://www.gwu.edu/~action/2008/adso8p /newspadsint.html#hc. Accessed January 2, 2012.

Anderson, Richard. "Defending the Practice of Medicine." *Archives of Internal Medicine* 164, no. 11 (2004): 1173–78.

Arrow, Kenneth, and William Capron. "Dynamic Shortages and Price Rises: The Engineer-Scientist Case." *Quarterly Journal of Economics* 73, no. 2 (1959): 292–308.

Baucus, Max. "Doctors, Patients, and the Need for Health Care Reform." *New England Journal of Medicine* 361 (November 5, 2009): 1817–19.

Beauchamp, Dan E. *Health Care Reform and the Battle for the Body Politic.* Philadelphia: Temple University Press, 1996.

Berliner, Howard, and Eli Ginsberg. "Why This Hospital Nursing Shortage Is Different." *Journal of the American Medical Association* 288, no. 21 (2002): 2742–44.

Best, Joel. *Random Violence: How We Talk About New Crimes and New Victims.* Berkeley and Los Angeles: University of California Press, 1999.

Blendon, Robert J., and John Benson. "Americans' Views on Health Policy: A Fifty-Year Historical Perspective." *Health Affairs* 20, no. 2 (2001): 33–46.

———. "Understanding How Americans View Health Care Reform." *New England Journal of Medicine* 361 (August 27, 2009): e13.

Blendon, Robert J., et al. "Americans' Health Priorities: Curing Cancer and Controlling Costs." *Health Affairs* 20, no. 6 (2001): 222–32.

Blumenthal, David. "Health Care Reform at the Close of the 20th Century." *New England Journal of Medicine* 340, no. 24 (1999): 1916–20.

Boorstin, Daniel. *The Image.* New York: Atheneum, 1962.

Bovbjerg, Randall. "Medical Malpractice: Folklore, Facts, and the Future." *Annals of Internal Medicine* 117, no. 9 (1992): 788–91.

Boyle, Ryan. "A Red Moon over the Mall: The Sputnik Panic and Domestic America." *Journal of American Culture* 31, no. 4 (2008): 373–82.

Brodie, Mollyann, et al. "Communicating Health Information Through the Entertainment Media." *Health Affairs* 20, no. 1 (2001): 192–200.

Brown, Lawrence. "The Amazing, Non-collapsing U.S. Health Care System: Is Reform Finally at Hand?" *New England Journal of Medicine* 358, no. 4 (2008): 325–27.

———. "Comparing Health Systems in Four Countries: Lessons for the United States." *American Journal of Public Health* 93, no. 1 (2003): 52–56.

Bush, George W. "Health Care Coverage and Drug Costs: The Candidates Speak Out." *New England Journal of Medicine* 351, no. 18 (2004): 1815–19.

———. "Remarks at High Point University in High Point, North Carolina." *Weekly Compilation of Presidential Documents*, July 25, 2002.

Callahan, Daniel. "Cost Control: Time to Get Serious." *New England Journal of Medicine* 361, no. 1 (2009): e10.

Charon, Rita. "Narrative Medicine: A Model for Empathy, Reflection, Profession, and Trust." *Journal of the American Medical Association* 286, no. 15 (2001): 1897–1902.

Cheng, Tsung-mei, and Uwe Reinhart. "The Ethics of America's Health Care Debate." In *Uniting America: Restoring the Vital Center to American Democracy*, edited by Norman Garfinkle and Daniel Yankelovich. New Haven, CT: Yale University Press, 2005.

Chesterton, G. K. *What's Wrong with the World?* 1910. http://www.gutenberg.org /files/1717/1717-h/1717-h.htm.

Clinton, Hillary. "Remarks on American Health Choices Plan." September 18, 2007. http://www.realclearpolitics.com/articles/2007/09/remarks_on_american _health_cho.html.

Clinton, Hillary Rodham, and Barack Obama. "Making Patient Safety the Centerpiece of Medical Liability Reform." *New England Journal of Medicine* 354, no. 21 (2006): 2205–8.

Clinton, William J. "Address Before a Joint Session of Congress." September 22, 1993. http://www.ibiblio.org/nhs/supporting/remarks.html.

———. "Address Before a Joint Session of the Congress on the State of the Union." January 25, 1994. http://www.presidency.ucsb.edu/ws/?pid=50409.

———. "Letter to Congressional Leaders on the 'Health Security Act of 1993.'" *Weekly Compilation of Presidential Documents*, October 27, 1993.

———. "Remarks in the ABC News *Nightline* Town Meeting in Tampa, Florida." *Presidential Papers*, September 23, 1993, 1863.

Cobb, Roger W., and Charles Elder. *Participation in American Politics*. 2nd ed. Baltimore: Johns Hopkins University Press, 1983.

Colby, David C., and Timothy Cook. "Epidemics and Agendas: The Politics of Nightly News Coverage of AIDS." *Journal of Health Politics, Policy, and Law* 16, no. 2 (1991): 215–49.

Corbett, Sara. "The Last Shift." *New York Times Magazine*, March 16, 2003, 58–61.

Cowley, Geoffrey. "The Future of Medicine." In "Your Health in the 21st Century." Special issue, *Newsweek*, Summer 2005, 9.

Crichton, Michael. "The High Cost of Cure." *Atlantic Monthly*, March 1970. http://www .theatlantic.com/past/unbound/flashbks/health/crichton.htm.

Danzon, Patricia. "The Frequency and Severity of Medical Malpractice Claims." *Journal of Law and Economics* 27, no. 1 (1984): 115–48.

DeNavas-Walt, Carmen, Bernadette D. Proctor, and Cheryl Hill Lee, US Census Bureau. *Current Population Reports, P60-231, Income, Poverty, and Health Insur-*

ance Coverage in the United States: 2005. Washington, DC: US Government Printing Office, 2006.

Denby, David. "Calculating Rhythm." *New Yorker,* March 4, 2002, 90–91.

Disch, Linda. "Publicity-Stunt Participation and Sound Bite Polemics: The Health Care Debate, 1993–94." *Journal of Health Politics, Policy, and Law* 21, no. 1 (1996): 3–33.

Dokupil, Tony. "When Nurses Strike in New York." *Newsweek,* May 3, 2010, 8.

Donelan, Karen, Peter Buerhaus, Beth Ulrich, Linda Norman, and Robert Dittus. "Awareness and Perceptions of the Johnson and Johnson Campaign for Nursing's Future: Views from Nursing Students, RNs, and CNOs." *Nursing Economics* 23 (July–August 2005): 151.

Duke, Paul. "If ER Nurses Crash, Will Patients Follow?" *Newsweek,* February 2, 2004, 12.

Edelman, Murray. *Constructing the Political Spectacle.* Chicago: University of Chicago Press, 1988.

———. *The Symbolic Uses of Politics.* Urbana: University of Illinois Press, 1964.

Edwards, John. "Press Release: Edwards Announces Plan for Universal Health Care." February 5, 2007. http://www.presidency.ucsb.edu/ws/?pid=93834.

Eisenberg, Daniel, and Maggie Sieger. "The Doctor Won't See You Now." *Time,* June 9, 2003.

Eisenhower, Dwight D. "Farewell Address to the American People." 1961. http://www.ourdocuments.gov/doc.php?flash=true&doc=90&page=transcript.

Fein, Rashi. "Social and Economic Attitudes Shaping American Health Care Policy." *Milbank Memorial Fund Quarterly: Health and Society* 58, no. 3 (1980): 349–85.

Ferraro, Geraldine. "How to Mend a Sick System." *Newsweek,* October 29, 2007, 66.

Fiorina, Morris. *Disconnect: The Breakdown of Representation in American Politics.* Norman: University of Oklahoma Press, 2009.

Fiorina, Morris, Samuel Abrams, and Jeremy Pope. "Polarization in the American Public: Misconceptions and Misreadings." *Journal of Politics* 70, no. 3 (2008): 556–60.

Fisher, Walter. *Human Communication as Narration.* Columbia: University of South Carolina Press, 1987.

Frank, Richard G. "Prescription Drug Prices." *New England Journal of Medicine* 351, no. 14 (2004): 1375–77.

Frist, William. "Health Care in the 21st Century." *New England Journal of Medicine* 352, no. 3 (2005): 267–72.

Fuchs, Victor R. "The Growing Demand for Medical Care." *New England Journal of Medicine* 279 (1968): 190–95.

Gabel, Jon, Howard Cohen, and Steven Fink. "Americans' Views on Health Care: Foolish Inconsistencies?" *Health Affairs* 8, no. 1 (1989): 103–18.

Gauthier, Candace Cummins. "Television Drama and Popular Film as Medical Narrative." *Journal of American Culture* 22, no. 1 (1999): 23–25.

Gawande, Atul. *The Checklist Manifesto.* New York: Metropolitan Books, 2009.

———. *Complications.* New York: Picador, 2003.

———."Getting There from Here: How Should Obama Reform Health Care?" *New Yorker,* January 26, 2009.

———. "Now What?" *New Yorker,* April 5, 2010, 21.

Ginsberg, Eli. "Health Care Reform: Why So Slow?" *New England Journal of Medicine* 322, no. 20 (1990): 1464–66.

Ginsberg, Paul B. "Controlling Health Care Costs." *New England Journal of Medicine* 351, no. 16 (2004): 1591–93.

Gordon, Suzanne. "What Nurses Stand For." *Atlantic Monthly,* February 1997, 87–88.

Gordon, Suzanne, and Bernice Buresh. "Doc Hollywood." *American Prospect,* May 21, 2001, 34.

Gostin, Lawrence. "A Public Health Approach to Reducing Error." *Journal of the American Medical Association* 283, no. 13 (2000): 1742–43.

Grassley, Chuck. "Health Care Reform: A Republican View." *New England Journal of Medicine* 361, no. 25 (2009): 2397–99.

Hacker, P. M. S. *Wittgenstein.* New York: Routledge, 1999.

Hackey, Robert B. "Symbolic Politics and Health Care Reform in the 1940s and 1990s." In *Cultural Strategies of Agenda Denial,* edited by Roger Cobb and Marc H. Ross, 141–57. Lawrence: University Press of Kansas, 1997.

Halberstam, Michael J. "The Doctor's New Dilemma: 'Will I Be Sued?'" *New York Times Magazine,* February 14, 1971.

Hanft, Ruth S. "National Health Expenditures, 1950–65." *Social Security Bulletin* 30, no. 2 (1967): 3–13.

Hart, Roderick P., and Susan Daughton. *Modern Rhetorical Criticism.* 3rd ed. Boston: Allyn and Bacon, 2004.

Hart, Roderick P., Sharon Jarvis, William P. Jennings, and Deborah Smith-Howell. *Political Keywords: Using Language That Uses Us.* New York: Oxford University Press, 2005.

Hatch, Orrin. "The Medical Malpractice Crisis: Physicians' Concern over Future Liability Costs Is Adversely Affecting Access to Health Care for All Americans." *Roll Call,* March 26, 1990.

Hertzberg, Hendrick. "Come Together." *New Yorker,* March 8, 2010, 19.

———. "Electoral Dissonance." *New Yorker,* November 15, 2010, 31–32.

———. "Ghostbusters." *New Yorker,* October 1, 2007, 38–39.

———. "Lies." *New Yorker,* September 21, 2009, 33–34.

———. "Tuesday, and After." *New Yorker,* September 24, 2001.

Hirschman, Albert O. *Exit, Voice, and Loyalty: Responses to Decline in Firms, Organizations, and States.* Cambridge, MA: Harvard University Press, 1970.

———. *The Rhetoric of Reaction.* Cambridge, MA: Belknap Press, 1990.

———. *Shifting Involvements.* Princeton, NJ: Princeton University Press, 1983.

Hodgson, Godfrey. *America in Our Time.* New York: Vintage, 1978.

———. "The Politics of American Health Care: What Is It Costing You?" *Atlantic Monthly,* October 1973, 45–61.

Hoffman, Beatrix. "Health Care Reform and Social Movements in the United States." *American Journal of Public Health* 93, no. 1 (2003): 75–85.

————. *The Wages of Sickness.* Chapel Hill: University of North Carolina Press, 2001.

Hollander, John. "Fear Itself." *Social Research* 71, no. 4 (2004): 865–86.

Huntington, Samuel. *American Politics: The Promise of Disharmony.* Cambridge, MA: Belknap Press, 1981.

————. "The United States." In *The Crisis of Democracy: Report on the Governability of Democracies to the Trilateral Commission.* New York: New York University Press, 1973. http://www.trilateral.org/download/doc/crisis_of_democracy.pdf.

Hyman, David A., and Charles Silver. "Believing Six Improbable Things: Medical Malpractice and 'Legal Fear.'" *Harvard Journal of Law and Public Policy* 28, no. 1 (2004): 107–18.

Iglehart, John. "The American Health Care System: Expenditures." *New England Journal of Medicine* 340, no. 1 (1999): 70–76.

————. "Historic Passage: Reform at Last." *New England Journal of Medicine* 362, no. 14 (2010): e48.

Institute of Medicine. *To Err Is Human: Building a Safer Health Care System.* Washington, DC: National Academy Press, 2000.

Jacobs, Lawrence R. "Health Reform Impasse: The Politics of American Ambivalence Toward Government." *Journal of Health Politics, Policy, and Law* 18, no. 3 (1993): 629–55.

————. "1994 All over Again? Public Opinion and Health Care." *New England Journal of Medicine* 358, no. 18 (2008): 1881–83.

Jacobs, Lawrence R., Robert Shapiro, and Eli Shulman. "Medical Care in the United States: An Update." *Public Opinion Quarterly* 57, no. 3 (1993): 394–427.

Jajich-Toth, Cindy, and Burns W. Roper. "Americans' Views on Health Care: A Study in Contradictions." *Health Affairs* 9, no. 4 (1990): 149–57.

Joint Commission on the Accreditation of Healthcare Organizations. *Health Care at the Crossroads: Strategies for Addressing the Evolving Nursing Crisis.* 2002. http://www.jointcommission.org/assets/1/18/health_care_at_the_crossroads.pdf.

Jones, Roger. "Analytic Philosophy." http://www.philosopher.org.uk/anal.htm Accessed December 27, 2011.

Kaiser Family Foundation. *Kaiser Health Tracking Poll: December 2010.* December 2010. http://www.kff.org/kaiserpolls/upload/8127-C.pdf.

————. *Kaiser Health Tracking Poll: December 2011.* December 2011. http://kff.org/kaiserpolls/upload/8265-C.pdf.

Keaney, Laura. "Examining Medical Error: Causes, Consequences, and Checklists." Unpublished manuscript, 2011.

Kennedy, Edward M. *In Critical Condition: The Crisis in America's Health Care.* New York: Simon and Schuster, 1972.

Kerrey, Bob. "Remarks to the National Newspaper Association Government Affairs Conference." Washington, DC, March 14, 1991. http://www.c-spanvideo.org/program/17080-1.

Kerry, John. "Health Care for All Americans." Speech delivered in Faneuil Hall, Boston, July 31, 2006. http://blog.thedemocraticdaily.com/?p=3759.

Kimball, Bobbi, and Edward O'Neil. "The Evolution of a Crisis: Nursing in America." *Politics, Policy, and Nursing Practice* 2, no. 3 (2001): 180–86.

———. *Health Care's Human Crisis: The American Nursing Shortage.* Robert Wood Johnson Foundation, April 2002. http://www.rwjf.org/files/newsroom/NursingReport.pdf.

Kissick, William L. "Health Policy Directions for the 1970s." *New England Journal of Medicine* 282 (June 11, 1970): 1343–54.

Klatch, Rebecca. "Of Meanings and Masters: Political Symbolism and Symbolic Action." *Polity* 21, no. 1 (1988): 137–54.

Klein, Burton. "The Limits to Growth: A Report for the Club of Rome." Social Science Working Paper 92. Pasadena: California Institute of Technology, 1975. http://www.hss.caltech.edu/SSPapers/sswp92.pdf.

Korcok, Milan. "'Perfect Storm' Brewing in US Because of Nursing Shortage." *Canadian Medical Association Journal* 167, no. 10 (2002): 1159.

Kotelchuck, David. "The Health Status of Americans." In *Prognosis Negative,* edited by David Kotelchuck, 5–20. New York: Vintage, 1976.

Kotlikoff, Laurence. *The Healthcare Fix.* Cambridge: MIT Press, 2007.

Kuehn, Bridget. "No End in Sight to Nursing Shortage." *Journal of the American Medical Association* 298, no. 14 (2007): 1623–25.

Kuklick, Bruce. *The Good Ruler: From Herbert Hoover to Richard Nixon.* New Brunswick, NJ: Rutgers University Press, 1988.

Ladd, Everett C. "The Congress Problem." *Public Interest* 100 (Summer 1990): 57–67.

Langston, Thomas. *With Reverence and Contempt.* Baltimore: Johns Hopkins University Press, 1995.

Lave, Judith R., and Lester Lave. *The Hospital Construction Act: An Evaluation of the Hill-Burton Program, 1948–1973.* Washington, DC: American Enterprise Institute, 1974.

Leape, Lucian, et al. "Promoting Patient Safety by Preventing Medical Error." *Journal of the American Medical Association* 280, no. 16 (1998): 1444–47.

Lemann, Nicholas. "Kennedy Care." *New Yorker,* September 7, 2009, 22.

Liang, Bryan. "Risks of Reporting Sentinel Events." *Health Affairs* 19, no. 5 (2000): 112–20.

Light, Donald. "Sociological Perspectives on Competition in Health Care." *Journal of Health Politics, Policy, and Law* 25, no. 5 (2000): 969–74.

Lundberg, George. "National Health Care Reform: An Aura of Inevitability Is upon Us." *Journal of the American Medical Association* 265, no. 19 (1991): 2566–67.

Madison, George W., et al. "Brief for Petitioners (Minimum Coverage Provision) No. 11-398 Submitted to the Supreme Court of the United States, Re: *Department of Health and Human Services et al. v. State of Florida et al.*" http://www.thehill.com/images/stories/blogs/healthwatch/dojbrief.pdf. Accessed January 8, 2012.

Mangan, Katherine S. "The Malpractice Menace." *Chronicle of Higher Education* (September 19, 2003): A16.

Marmor, Theodore R. "A Summer of Discontent: Press Coverage of Murder and Medical Care Reform." *Journal of Health Politics, Policy, and Law* 20, no. 2 (1995): 495–501.

Matthiessen, Constance. "Bordering on Collapse." *Modern Maturity,* October–November 1990.

McCain, John. "Remarks at a Town Hall Meeting in Sun City, Arizona." *CQ Transcriptions* (August 25, 2009).

McCaughey, Elizabeth. "No Exit." *New Republic,* February 7, 1994, 21–25.

McConnell, Grant. *Private Power and American Democracy.* New York: Alfred A. Knopf, 1966.

Mechanic, David. "Some Dilemmas in Health Care Policy." *Milbank Memorial Fund Quarterly: Health and Society* 59, no. 1 (1981): 1–15.

Mello, Michelle. "Managing Malpractice Crises." *Journal of Law, Medicine, and Ethics* 33, no. 3 (2005): 414–15.

Mello, Michelle, and Thomas Gallagher. "Malpractice Reform: Opportunities for Leadership by Health Care Institutions and Liability Insurers." *New England Journal of Medicine* 362, no. 15 (2010): 1353–56.

Mello, Michelle, David Studdert, and Troyen Brennan. "The New Medical Malpractice Crisis." *New England Journal of Medicine* 348, no. 23 (2003): 2281–84.

Mohr, James C. "American Medical Malpractice Litigation in Historical Perspective." *Journal of the American Medical Association* 283, no. 13 (2000): 1731–37.

Mongan, James, and Thomas Lee. "Do We Really Want Broad Access to Health Care?" *New England Journal of Medicine* 352, no. 12 (2005): 1260–63.

Morone, James A. *The Democratic Wish.* New York: Basic Books, 1990.

———. "Nativism, Hollow Corporations, and Managed Competition: Why the Clinton Health Care Reform Failed." *Journal of Health Politics, Policy, and Law* 20, no. 2 (1995): 391–98.

Morris, Charles. *Too Much of a Good Thing? Why Health Care Spending Won't Make Us Sick.* New York: Century Fund, 2000.

Nichols, Len. "Be Not Afraid." *New England Journal of Medicine* 362, no. 1 (2010): e30.

Nixon, Richard M. "Remarks at a Briefing on the Nation's Health System." *Weekly Compilation of Presidential Documents,* July 10, 1969, 964.

Nye, David. *Narratives and Spaces: Technology and the Construction of American Culture.* New York: Columbia University Press, 1998.

Obama, Barack. "Cutting Costs and Covering America: A 21st Century Health Care System." Remarks delivered at the University of Iowa, Iowa City, May 29, 2007. http://www-958.ibm.com/software/data/cognos/manyeyes/datasets/cutting-costs-and-covering-america/versions/1.txt.

———. "Remarks by the President at Signing of Children's Health Insurance Program Legislation." February 4, 2009. http://www.whitehouse.gov/blog_post/covering_kids/.

———. "Transcript of Address to the 2009 Annual Meeting of the AMA House of Delegates." Hyatt Regency Hotel, Chicago, June 15, 2009. http://www.whitehouse.gov/the_press_office/Remarks-by-the-President-to-the-Annual-Conference-of-the-American-Medical-Association.

———. *Weekly Radio Address* (June 13, 2009). http://www.whitehouse.gov/the_press_office/Weekly-Address-and-Fact-Sheet-New-Savings-Announcement.

Oberlander, Jonathan. "Beyond Repeal: The Future of Health Care Reform." *New England Journal of Medicine* 363, no. 24 (2010): 2277–79.

————. "The Politics of Health Reform: Why Do Bad Things Happen to Good Plans?" *Health Affairs.* August 27, 2003. http://content.healthaffairs.org/content /early/2003/08/27/hlthaff.w3.391.citation.

O'Connor, Michael M. "The Role of the Television Drama *ER* in Medical Student Life: Entertainment or Socialization?" *Medical Student JAMA* 280, no. 9 (1998): 854–55.

Ohmann, Richard. "In Lieu of a New Rhetoric." *College English* 26 (October 1964): 17–22.

Orwell, George. "Politics and the English Language." *Horizon* (April 1946). http://www .mtholyoke.edu/acad/intrel/orwell46.htm.

Palmisano, Donald J. "Why Your Doctor Might Quit." *Saturday Evening Post,* November–December 2004, 50.

Perlstein, Rick. *Nixonland.* New York: Scribner, 2008.

Piccola, Jeffrey. "Cap Noneconomic Damages, Attorneys' Fees." *Physician News Digest* (June 2003). http://www.physiciansnews.com/commentary/603piccola.html.

Quaid, Dennis, Julie Thao, and Charles Denham. "Story Power: The Secret Weapon." *Journal of Patient Safety* 6, no. 1 (2010): 5–14.

Reason, James T. "Human Error: Models and Management." *British Medical Journal* 320 (2000): 768–70.

Reinhardt, Uwe. "Wanted: A Clearly Articulated Social Ethic for American Health Care." *Journal of the American Medical Association* 278, no. 17 (1997): 1446–47.

Rideout, Victoria. *Television as a Health Educator: A Case Study of "Grey's Anatomy."* Menlo Park, CA: Henry J. Kaiser Family Foundation, 2008. http://www.kff.org /entmedia/upload/7803.pdf.

Roberts-Miller, Patricia. "Democracy, Demagoguery, and Critical Rhetoric." *Rhetoric and Public Affairs* 8, no. 3 (2005): 459–76.

Robinson, Glen O. "The Medical Malpractice Crisis of the 1970s: A Retrospective." *Law and Contemporary Problems* 49 (Spring 1986): 7–8.

Rodgers, Daniel T. *Contested Truths: Keywords in American Politics Since Independence.* New York: Basic Books, 1987.

Rosenbaum, Sara. "The Impact of United States Law on Medicine as a Profession." *Journal of the American Medical Association* 289, no. 12 (2003): 1546–55.

Rosenblatt, Stanley. "In His Own Words." *People,* October 9, 1978, 112.

Rothman, David J. *Beginnings Count: The Technological Imperative in American Health Care.* New York: Oxford University Press, 1997.

————. "A Century of Failure: Health Care Reform in America." *Journal of Health Politics, Policy, and Law* 18, no. 2 (1993): 271–86.

Rotunda, Ronald. *The Politics of Language.* Iowa City: University of Iowa Press, 1986.

Rovner, Julie. "'Play or Pay' Gains Momentum as Labor Panel Marks Up Bill." *Congressional Quarterly Weekly Report* (January 25, 1992): 172–74.

Saad, Sydia. "No Increase in Public Pressure for Healthcare Reform." Gallup Poll, November 29, 2007. http://www.gallup.com/poll/102931/increase-public-pressure -healthcare-reform.aspx.

Sadusk, Joseph F. "Hazardous Fields of Medicine in Relation to Professional Liability." *Journal of the American Medical Association* 163, no. 11 (1957): 953–57.

Samuelson, Robert J. "Obama's Unhealthy Choices." *Newsweek*, January 11, 2009.

Sandor, Andrew. "The History of Professional Liability Suits in the United States." *Journal of the American Medical Association* 163, no. 6 (1957): 459–66.

Schoenbaum, Stephen C., and Randall Bovbjerg. "Malpractice Reform Must Include Steps to Prevent Medical Injury." *Annals of Internal Medicine* 140, no. 1 (2004): 51–53.

Schram, Sanford, and Philip Neisser. Introduction to *Tales of the State: Narrative in Contemporary U.S. Politics and Public Policy*, edited by S. Schram and P. Neisser. Lanham, MD: Rowman and Littlefield, 1997.

Schwartz, William. *Life Without Disease: The Pursuit of Medical Utopia*. Berkeley and Los Angeles: University of California Press, 1998.

Shmanske, Stephen, and Tina Stevens. "The Performance of Medical Malpractice Review Panels." *Journal of Health Politics, Policy, and Law* 11, no. 3 (1986): 525–35.

Shortell, Stephen, and Walter McNerney. "Criteria and Guidelines for Reforming the U.S. Health Care System." *New England Journal of Medicine* 322, no. 7 (1990): 463–67.

Sloan, Frank. "State Responses to the Malpractice Insurance 'Crisis' of the 1970s: An Empirical Assessment." *Journal of Health Politics, Policy, and Law* 9, no. 4 (1985): 629–46.

Smeltzer, Carolyn Hope, Frances Vlasses, and Connie Robinson. "'If We Only Had a Nurse' . . . Historical View of a Nurse Shortage." *Journal of Nursing Care Quality* 20, no. 2 (2005): 191.

Sobel, Lester, ed. "Malpractice Dilemma." In *Health Care: An American Crisis*, edited by L. Sobel. New York: Facts on File, 1976.

Somers, Herman M., and Anne R. Somers. *Doctors, Patients, and Health Insurance*. New York: Anchor Books, 1961.

Sowell, Thomas. "Memo to Medical Reformers." *Forbes*, June 21, 1993, 140.

Starr, Paul. "The Lost Crusade." *American Prospect*, February 14, 2000, 6.

Steckel, Richard. "Hospitals and Beds, by Type of Hospital: 1946–1997." Table Bd118-131 in *Historical Statistics of the United States: Earliest Times to the Present*, edited by Susan Carter et al. Vol. 2. Pt. B, "Work and Welfare." Millennial Edition. New York: Cambridge University Press.

Steinbrook, Robert. "Nursing in the Crossfire." *New England Journal of Medicine* 346, no. 22 (2002): 1757–66.

Stone, Deborah. *Policy Paradox: The Art of Political Decision Making*. New York: W. W. Norton, 1997.

Stone, Deborah, and Theodore Marmor. "Introduction." *Journal of Health Politics, Policy, and Law* 15, no. 2 (1990): 253–57.

Studdert, David, Michelle Mello, and Troyen Brennan. "Medical Malpractice." *New England Journal of Medicine* 350, no. 3 (2004): 283–92.

Studdert, David, et al. "Defensive Medicine Among High-Risk Specialist Physicians in a Volatile Malpractice Environment." *Journal of the American Medical Association* 293, no. 21 (2005): 2609–17.

Sundquist, James. "The Crisis of Competence in Our National Government." *Political Science Quarterly* 95, no. 2 (1980): 183–208.

Taylor, Humphrey, and Robert Leitman. "Attitudes Towards the United States' Health Care System: Long-Term Trends." *Health Care News* 2 (August 21, 2002).

Thomas, Evan, and Stuart Taylor Jr. "Fight Club." *Newsweek,* January 11, 2010, 48–49.

Trust for America's Health. "Nursing Shortage Estimates (2010)." http://healthyamericans.org/states/states.php?measure=nursingshortage. Accessed December 27, 2011.

Turow, Joseph, and Rachel Gans. *As Seen on TV: Health Policy Issues in TV's Medical Dramas.* Menlo Park, CA: Henry J. Kaiser Family Foundation, 2002. http://www.kff .org/entmedia/John_Q_Report.pdf.

US Department of Health, Education, and Welfare. *Medical Malpractice: Report of the Secretary's Commission on Medical Malpractice.* Pub. No. 73-88. Washington, DC: US Government Printing Office, January 1973.

US Department of Labor. Bureau of Labor Statistics. *Occupational Outlook Handbook.* http://www.bls.gov/oco/. Accessed December 24, 2011.

Vladeck, Bruce. "Universal Health Insurance in the United States: Reflections on the Past, the Present, and the Future." *American Journal of Public Health* 93, no. 1 (2003): 16–19.

Waldman, Allison. "Dramas Deliver Medical Messages: Fiction Programming Can Create Awareness of Health Care, Diseases." *Television Week,* March 12, 2007, 20.

Wallack, Lawrence, and Regina Lawrence. "Talking About Public Health: Developing America's 'Second Language.'" *American Journal of Public Health* 95, no. 4 (2005): 567–70.

Webb, Kandy G. "Recent Medical Malpractice Legislation: A First Checkup." *Tulane Law Review* 50 (1976): 655–60.

Weintraub, Arline. "Nursing: On the Critical List." *Business Week,* June 3, 2002, 81.

West, Darrell M. *Congress and Economic Policymaking.* Pittsburgh: University of Pittsburgh Press, 1987.

Will, George. "Word Spill." *Newsweek,* June 28, 2010, 28.

Wooley, Mary, and Stacie Propst. "Public Attitudes and Perceptions About Health-Related Research." *Journal of the American Medical Association* 294, no. 11 (2005): 1380–84.

Woolf, Virginia. "Mr. Bennett and Mrs. Brown." http://stuttercut.org/165ML/Bennett _and_Brown.pdf. Accessed December 23, 2011.

Yankelovich, Daniel. "The Debate That Wasn't: The Public and the Clinton Health Care Plan." In *The Problem That Won't Go Away,* edited by Henry J. Aaron, 70–91. Washington, DC: Brookings Institution Press, 1995.

———. "Overcoming Polarization: The New Social Morality." In *Uniting America: Restoring the Vital Center to American Democracy,* edited by Norman Garfinkle and Daniel Yankelovich. New Haven, CT: Yale University Press, 2005.

Zakaria, Fareed. "America's Fatal Flaw." *Newsweek,* August 24, 2009, 26.

Zuckerman, Mortimer. "America's High Anxiety." *U.S. News and World Report,* December 25, 2006, 100.